The Computer Diet

Vincent W. Antonetti, PhD

NoPaperPress, LLC

Contents

1. INTRODUCTION
How It All Started (6)
Research (7)
Developing a Predictive Equation (9)
Verifying the Equations (9)
A Scientific Paper (11)
A Significant Update (11)
The Weight Control Tables (11)
What Is In This Book (12)

2. WEIGHT & ENERGETICS
Conservation of Energy (14)
When Weight Change Occurs (15)
Human Energy Constituents (15)
Activity Levels (16)

3. NUTRITION BASICS
Complete & Incomplete Proteins (18)
You Need Healthy Carbs (19)
Fat Facts (19)
You Need Fiber (21)
Eat Slowly (21)
Vitamins and Minerals (22)

4. EXERCISE BASICS
Select the Right Exercise (24)
Aerobic Exercise: How Hard? (25)
Get a Pedometer - Count Steps (26)
Strength-Building Programs (26)
Risks and Possible Problems (27)
Avoiding Injury (28)

5. ABOUT YOUR WEIGHT
What You Should Weigh (31)
Body Fat Percentage (33)

6. WEIGHT LOSS
Diet Options (34)

Example 1 (35)
Suppose Your Weight Isn't In Table? (36)
The Physiology of Weight Loss (36)
Weight Loss Principles (37)
Selecting a Weight Loss Diet (38)

7. WEIGHT MAINTENANCE
Why You Gain Weight With Age (39)
Why You Gain Weight After a Diet (40)
People Who Regained Lost Weight (40)
People Who Maintained Lost Weight (41)
Select Correct Weight Maintenance Table (41)
Example 2 (42)
Weight Maintenance is a Life-Long Struggle (42)
Get Off the Diet Roller Coaster (43)

8. SAMPLE WEIGHT LOSS & MAINTENANCE DIETS
Sample 1200 Calorie Daily Meal Plan (45)
Sample 1200 Calorie Recipe (46)
Sample 1500 Calorie Daily Meal Plan (47)
Sample 1500 Calorie Recipe (48)
Sample 1500 Calorie Daily Meal Plan (49)
Sample Weight Maintenance Daily Meal Plan (50)
Sample Weight Maintenance Recipe (51)

Appendix A Weight Loss Prediction Tables - Men (52)

Appendix B Weight Loss Prediction Tables - Women (89)

Appendix C Weight Maintenance Tables - Men (114)

Appendix D Weight Maintenance Tables - Women (124)

Appendix E Updated Weight Loss Predictive Model (131)

Appendix F Bibliography (136)

NoPaperPress Paperbacks & eBooks (137)

Disclaimer

The Author

Index of Tables

Table 1: Physical Activity Levels (17)
Table 2: Fats in Foods (20)
Table 3: RDA for Selected Vitamins (22)
Table 4: RDA for Selected Minerals (23)
Table 5: Caloric Cost of Various Activities (26)
Table 6: BMI-Based Weight vs. Height (32)
Table 7: Portion of Weight Loss Table B.1 (34)
Table 8: Sample 1200 Calorie Daily Meal Plan (45)
Table 9: Sample 1500 Calorie Daily Meal Plan (47)
Table 10: Sample 1500 Cal No-Cooking Meal Plan (49)
Table 11: Sample 2500 Cal Weight Maintenance Meal Plan (50)

Table AA: Index of 36 Weight Loss Prediction Tables - Men (52)
Table BB: Index of 24 Weight Loss Prediction Tables - Women (89)
Table CC: Index of 9 Weight Maintenance Tables - Men (114)
Table DD: Index of 6 Weight Maintenance Tables - Women (124)

1. Introduction

The original hard-cover book *The Computer Diet*, published in 1973, was very well received and critically acclaimed. But now portions of the book are out of date. So at the insistence of some researchers and nutritionists who still refer to the original book, I decided to write an updated version, and published it in a U.S. edition, as well as a first-time metric edition.

My interest in fitness, nutrition and eventually weight control started when I was twelve years old. My uncle, who was exactly ten years older than I was, had just been discharged from the U.S. Army. He decided to join a gym and I begged him to take me along. There were no fancy health clubs in those days – at least none that I knew of. The "gym" in reality was a converted three-car garage equipped with a pot belly stove. But inside there were some serious weight lifters. The members were not thrilled to have a twelve-year old kid in their midst. But the owner of the "gym" was an army buddy of my uncle, so he allowed me to join. He gave me a basic workout routine; stationed me in a corner and told me not to speak unless spoken to.

In that corner I did curls, presses, dead lifts, squats, shrugs, rows and got stronger. I also listened to the guys talk about what they ate and why they trained as they did. In due course I started to ask questions and got hooked on fitness and nutrition. I read every nutrition and exercise book in our local library. But after six months my family moved from an apartment to a one-family house with a detached-garage in the back, which I converted into a "gym" for myself and my new neighborhood friends.

How It All Started
Fast forward about twenty years. "We guarantee a weight loss of two pounds per week," read a newspaper advertisement sponsored by a weight control company. My wife wanted to lose ten pounds and decided to attend a meeting.

Later, as my wife and I discussed what had transpired at the meeting, she said, "There was one point that didn't make sense. When I asked how long I would continue to lose two pounds a week," the speaker answered, 'for as long as you stay on the diet.' "My wife laughed when I remarked, "That would mean one year on that diet and you would disappear!"

We both concluded that what must happen in time is that weight loss would taper off. I then asked if the same diet was suggested for everyone. "Yes," she replied, "and everyone is supposed to lose two pounds per week." I continued, "That really doesn't make sense. In effect what they are saying is: if you and, for example, a professional football player went on the same diet, both of you would lose weight at the same rate."

Intuitively, it seemed to me that if my wife and a 6' 3" 260 pound football player were on the same diet, the football player would practically be starving and would certainly lose more weight than would my wife.

At that time, I had stopped smoking and had promptly gained ten pounds. I was still gaining when I joined a YMCA. The exercise made me feel healthy and fit but I didn't lose weight.

As I recall, it was the conversation with my wife and my inability to lose weight that first aroused my interest in weight control. During the next five years, this casual interest grew into an after-hours research project, a literature search, a mathematical analysis, publication of a scientific paper, and in 1973 *The Computer Diet*.

Research
I began in the late 1960s by reading every diet book on the market. Frankly, I was not satisfied. The books were contradictory and because I am an engineer, I found they lacked the sort of quantitative information I was searching for. As a result, I gravitated toward the scientific literature. What I hoped to discover was a weight-loss predictive formula, or equation. I read books on physiology, nutrition, and then the latest research papers. And I found no such equation. I also began to correspond with scientists at leading universities.

My literature search revealed a tremendous amount of on-going weight control research but again no weight-loss predictive equation. There seemed to be two fundamentally different schools of thought concerning the nature of weight loss. One view argued that "calories do count," or in more scientific terms, that weight loss was governed by a fundamental concept of physics called the conservation of energy (which is discussed in greater detail in Chapter 2.) The contrary view, in brief, was that certain foods or food combinations had special qualities that cause weight to be lost more rapidly than would be predicted by the conservation of energy principle. I appraised both sides and the more deeply I read, the

7

more convinced I became that the "calories-do-count" faction had it right. It seemed perfectly reasonable to me that the human metabolism should obey the conservation of energy – as does everything else in nature! I further reasoned that if the conservation of energy applies to humans, it should be possible do a mathematical analysis of weight change in human beings. For years researchers have recognized that weight change depends on, at the very least, age, gender, height, weight, amount of physical activity, caloric intake and time. Unfortunately, the relationship of these factors to weight change had never been mathematically established. With the background in physiology and nutrition I had gained over the years through my reading, plus my engineering-mathematics training and experience, I set myself the task of developing the equations involved in weight change.

That I would attempt such an analysis is not as unusual as it might appear. There are a relatively large group of engineers working in a field that falls somewhere between medicine and engineering called bio-medical engineering. For years, these engineers have been developing advanced technology for use in medicine. Applications of engineering to medicine range from the development of cryogenic surgical instruments and electronic surveillance systems for hospitals to the design of prototype mechanical hearts.

In fact, engineers have devised mathematical models of various parts of the human body in order to better understand how they function. Such analyses include the application of engineering control theory to the function of the human brain and utilization of the principles of fluid mechanics to the study of the blood circulatory system. Moreover, any significant understanding of weight control requires a knowledge of the first law of thermodynamics as applied to humans. In fact, my particular engineering specialties, which are thermodynamics and heat transfer, were, therefore, particularly suited to this area of research.

Many of my friends were openly skeptical. "You can't do that. You can't analyze the human body as if were a machine!" My response was that the human body is a machine. The most complex and challenging machine I had ever analyzed. But I was sure that by taking the proper analytical approach, the weight change equations could be derived.

Developing a Predictive Equation

The analysis method I employed was not new. Engineers call the technique a generalized closed system approach. It has been used to solve many fundamental thermodynamic problems. In simple terms, the analysis is performed by considering the human body as a closed system, and recording what forms of energy and mass cross the system's boundary. Using this method, one is not concerned with what is happening inside the closed system, that is inside the human body. Only external energy and mass transformations are of importance. Once identified these quantities are related in accordance with the conservation of energy. As an analogy, the performance of a large and complex chemical process plant, with its maze of piping and equipment, is routinely understood and predicted by applying the conservation of energy to only the chemical streams entering and leaving the plant – without considering the internal reactions.

In the course of the development and verification of my weight change equations, certain physical, biological, medical and nutritional data were needed. In all cases, I obtained the necessary information from the latest and best available scientific sources.

When finished, my analysis produced the first and only weight change predictive equations in existence at that time. The equations represent a mathematical model of one facet of the human metabolism and provides a means to answer questions such as: How long will it take an individual of a given gender, age, height, weight, and activity level to lose a desired amount of weight when on a known diet? And how should one adjust his/her diet to maintain this lower weight?

Verifying the Equations

Once the weight change equations were derived, the next step was to verify, or validate, that they did indeed accurately predict weight change. There are essentially two ways to accomplish this. The first method involves setting up a series of experiments and observing the weight loss of a number of subjects. This technique would necessitate a research facility and would take years to accomplish. The second method would be to compare the theoretical predictions of my equations against weight loss data gathered over the years by various research teams. Of course, I decided on the latter method. Although there exists a great deal of weight loss experimental data in the literature, the most famous and comprehensive collection of data was gathered as part of what became known as The Minnesota Experiment. The time-frame was near the end of World War II. A team of research scientists at the Laboratory of Physiological Hygiene at the University of Minnesota had received reports from the U.S. government that starvation was widespread in the occupied countries of Europe and Asia, and in prisoner of war camps. There was a danger of a mass famine. It was apparent that at the end of hostilities the United States would be involved in a large-scale nutritional refeeding program. What was required – urgently – was a project to determine what changes occurred in humans due to semi-starvation and what would be the best sort of rehabilitation diet.

The subjects for the experiment were a volunteer group of U.S. conscientious objectors, who welcomed the opportunity to serve as human guinea pigs. The men were put on diets of approximately 1500 Calories per day for six months. And then they were re-nourished. The data from all phases of the program were recorded in a two-volume treatise entitled *The Biology of Human Starvation*. Among the myriad information gathered during the study was a tremendous amount of carefully documented weight loss data. I analyzed this data and found that my weight loss equation predicted the weight loss experienced by the conscientious objectors quite well.

But I did not stop checking. I compared the predictions of my weight change equation against other well-documented experiments conducted by research laboratories on male and female obese patients. In a variety of tests, patients were subjected to all types of diets – high fat, high protein, low carbohydrate, and so forth. As I suspected, the type of food eaten did not significantly alter my weight loss prediction. For a given subject, only the number of calories consumed appeared to be important. Now satisfied, I wrote a paper documenting my research.

At that time I was employed by IBM and managed an engineering department involved in the design of the first water-cooling system for large computers. Even though I worked on my weight change equations on my own time in the early morning and late at night, the result belonged to IBM. So I had to get IBM's permission to submit for possible publication the paper I called, "The Equations Governing Weight Change in Human Beings." To obtain IBM's permission required that the paper had to pass an internal IBM technical review. But none of the IBM engineers and scientists on the review committee felt they had the background and expertise to judge the paper. But they said they would approve my paper if I obtained the backing of a university professor in the field.

As it happened, I was already in touch with professor Francisco Grande a renowned researcher at the Laboratory of Physiological Hygiene at the University of Minnesota. He had already read my proposed paper and stated that, " ... the paper was a definite contribution to the literature." He later advised me to submit the paper to the *American Journal of Clinical Nutrition*. I didn't realize it at the time that he had been the editor of the AJCN for several years. Needless to say I had no problem getting the paper approved by IBM and then accepted by the AJCN.

A Scientific Paper
"The Equations Governing Weight Change in Human Beings" finally was published in the *American Journal of Clinical Nutrition*. In the paper the disciplines of mathematics, physiology and engineering are merged to establish the foundation for the first truly rational approach to weight control in humans.

A Significant Update
At the time that my weight-loss model was developed, the basil metabolic rate or the energy required to maintain the human body at rest was believed to best be represented by assuming it was dependent on body surface area. But this assumption made the resulting weight loss differential equation non-linear and required a relatively complex numerical solution using programmed software.

Then in 2016, professor of mathematics Diana Thomas of the U.S. Military Academy at West Point suggested that my original model be updated by replacing the resting metabolic rate portion of my model with a much newer, validated and widely used set of regression equations. As a bonus I found the update also eliminated the non-linearity in my original model and resulted in a differential equation with a much simpler closed-form solution, now called the Antonetti-Thomas weight loss model. This version of my original weight loss model was published in 2017 in chapter 12 of the book, *Advances in the Assessment of Dietary Intake* - published by CRC press.

The Weight Control Tables

"Appears quite logical and straightforward," said a chemist friend, after I showed him my original paper. "But," he continued, "it's not going to be used. The average medical doctor or dietician is not sufficiently skilled in math to apply your equations in practical weight control situations. Unless you translate your equations into a more practical form, you've wasted your time!" I realized my friend was right. Even in its simpler updated form, the latest version of my model was still considered too complex to be used by health care professionals. To apply the weight loss equations to a particular individual on a given diet, one would have to be proficient in advanced mathematics. Tables, I thought might be the answer. In tabular form the equations would be useful. Devising a tabular format was almost second nature to me. As a matter of fact, my colleagues at IBM and latter when I was a professor and chair of the mechanical engineering department at Manhattan College, often would often tease me because of my tendency to arrange virtually any set of data into a table. As you read on you will know what they meant.

In a short time, however, I understood that it would take me years to do the calculations needed to produce the tables I envisioned. It took me almost a half hour to compute just one number in the table and there were thousands of numbers to calculate! But using a computer, calculations of this scope are now commonplace. Luckily I had taught myself how to program early in my engineering career. The resulting tables are published in this book. These unique West Loss Prediction and Weight Maintenance tables make it possible for anyone to quickly determine the exact diet caloric intake needed to lose a given amount of weight, in a desired time frame, or to maintain a particular weight level.

What Is In This Book

In the following chapters, you are introduced to the relationship between weight control and energy. Next is a "cram course" in the basics of sensible nutrition and exercise. Then a new Activity Level Table is introduced and explained. Finally, the heart of the book, the unique Weight Loss Predictive and Weight Maintenance tables are presented. The use of these valuable, innovative tools in the development of a logical and personalized weight control plan is described.

For weight loss, there are 60 unique Weight Loss Prediction tables for men and women. In addition, there are sample 1200 and 1500 Calorie diets, all with sample no-cooking and cooking daily meal plans complete with delicious recipes.

Use the Weight Loss Prediction tables in conjunction with the Activity Level table, and the sample 1200 and 1500 Calorie weight loss meal plans to choose the diet calorie level that is best for you. Once you decide on your diet calorie level, you will be directed to NoPaperPress.com where you will find 7-Day, 30-Day, 60-Day, 90-Day and 100-Day (cooking and no-cooking) diets in eBook format. (Note that recently some of the eBooks have also been published as paperbacks.)

For weight maintenance, there are 15 Weight Maintenance tables for men and women, and a sample 2500 Calorie weight maintenance meal plan.

Use the Weight Maintenance tables in conjunction with the Activity Level table, and the sample 2500 Calorie weight maintenance meal plan to estimate how much you will be able to eat and still maintain your lost weight. (2500 Calories is a typical maintenance calorie level for a relatively inactive 45-year-old, 160 pound man). If you want more information, you will be directed to NoPaperPress.com where you will find *Weight Maintenance - U.S. Edition*, widely considered the best weight maintenance book available.

Finally, the last appendix at the end of this book contains a pertinent Bibliography.

2. Weight and Energetics

All human life depends on energy. Plants convert solar energy into chemical energy by a process called photosynthesis. The chemical energy is then used by plants to make carbohydrates, proteins and fats. We need energy to operate our body, but we cannot use solar energy directly. Instead we get the energy we need from the chemical energy contained in plants or other animals. When we eat food containing carbohydrates, proteins and fats, they are oxidized producing energy, carbon dioxide, water – and heat. This chapter contains a brief discussion of energy, as it generally pertains to our body and how energy relates to weight control.

Conservation of Energy

One of the greatest scientific achievements of the nineteenth century was the recognition and statement of the principle of conservation of energy by Julius Robert Von Mayer, in a classic paper that appeared in 1842 in Liebig's *Annalen der Chemie*. The principle is an inductive generalization based on observation of physical phenomenon and states that energy may be converted or transferred but cannot be created or destroyed. Then in 1847, Von Helmholtz, a surgeon in the Prussian army, wrote a brilliant paper applying the conservation of energy principle to the sciences of physiology and chemistry. By the beginning of the twentieth century, the scientific observations of Rubner, and then Atwater and Benedict, had demonstrated the validity of the law of the conservation of energy for the human metabolism.

According to the law of conservation of energy – as related to humans – the energy value of the food eaten (minus the energy lost in waste) must equal the sum of the heat energy leaving the body plus the physical work done by the body. In weight control, the measure of energy is the Calorie. Both the energy value of the food we eat and the energy we expend in day-to-day activities are expressed in terms of the Calorie. Another way of stating the conservation of energy as related to humans is: Weight is lost when the calories in the food one eats are less than calories one burns in physical activity. This is called a calorie deficit. And the calorie deficit is the driving force for weight loss.

An overwhelming number of scientists today agree that weight change in human beings is linked to their energy balance (or imbalance), and that

weight loss in humans is governed by the law of the conservation of energy.

When Weight Change Occurs
Simply stated, the generally accepted theory is that weight loss in human beings occurs when the energy expended by the body is greater the energy value of the food consumed. When this condition happens an energy imbalance occurs. In order to return to a state of energy balance, the body compensates by "burning" stored body weight, – mainly fat – which results in the liberation of energy. The net effect of this process is a loss of weight and the return of the body to an energy balance or equilibrium, in accord with conservation of energy. Weight gain can be explained by the converse of this reasoning.

Since weight is only lost or gained when there is an energy imbalance, the is no weight change when the energy value of the food eaten equals the amount of energy required by the body to maintain its present weight.

Human Energy Constituents
How much energy does a human being need? To answer this question, one must be aware of the energy constituents that comprise the body's total needs. The energy requirement of an adult human being is made up of three parts:

1. Basal (or resting) Energy: is that energy that is expended performing the body's involuntary basal processes. These processes include circulation, respiration, glandular activity, operation of the kidneys, and contractions of the intestines, etc., all of which consume energy. Scientists determine the basal energy by a carefully controlled test in which measurements are made on a subject that lies quietly and completely relaxed. Test results demonstrate that the basal metabolic energy is dependent on gender, age, height and weight, and that most individuals vary within plus or minus ten percent of what is considered normal.

2. Ingestive Energy: In a classic experiment in calorimetry, the famous French scientist Lavoisier discovered that the ingestion of food caused an increase in the heat produced by the body. This heat increase is due to the physical work involved in the mastication, digestion, and elimination of the food. This process is called the influence of food or specific dynamic action.

15

Ingestive energy was taken into account in deriving the weight control equations and tables in this book.

Another factor which influences the amount of energy expended by humans is the ambient or environmental temperature. But the effect of the ambient temperature is negligible in temperate zones where people are well clothed and homes are well heated.

3. Physical Activity Energy: As soon as one begins to move about, the physical activity causes energy expenditure to increase significantly above the basal level. Many experiments have been performed to determine the energy equivalent of various activities. Test results are usually listed in terms of calories per pound of body weight per unit of time. Thus to compute one's total energy due to physical activity, a diary of the amount of time spent at each activity must be kept for an entire day. The total activity energy would then be calculated by multiplying the amount of time spent at each activity by the caloric value per unit of time for each activity. The activity level for a given individual may be established after measuring the activity energy expended for perhaps ten days and averaging the result.

Activity Levels
Obviously such a determination would in most cases be impractical. Because of this I developed a new and more accessible parameter called the Activity Level. Essentially to use the Activity Level Method, you make a judgment of your physically activity energy expenditure using Table 1 on the following page as a guide.

It should be kept in mind that modern technology has, for most people, reduced physical demands, and that most people today are not as active as their ancestors.

- **Average American male is between Activity Levels 1 and 2.**
- **Average American female probably belongs in Activity Level 1.**

To determine your Activity Level will, in most cases, require considerable judgment on your part. As an aid, Table 1 matches the five Lifestyle Activity Levels to walking distances and an equivalent number of pedometer steps. Choose the option that best approximates the activity of your average day.

Activity Level	Lifestyle	Description	Equivalent Pedometer Steps
0	Sedentary	Inactive most of day. Stands & walks very little during the day.	Less than 3000
1	Relatively Inactive	Seated most of day. Stands & walks at most four hours. Typical of office workers & similar occupations.	About 5000
2	Moderately Active	Stands as often as is seated. Typical of teachers, sales clerks, & similar jobs.	About 8000
3	Very Active	Stands & walks most of day. Typical of factory & construction workers, farmers, & similar jobs.	About 11000
4	Extremely Active	Very hard physical work. Typical of lumber jacks, athletes in training, etc.	17,000 or more

Table 1: Lifestyle Activity Levels

3. Nutrition Basics

Healthy eating habits, the result of sensible nutritional practices, should be an integral part of any weight control program. Foods are made up of seven basic constituents: carbohydrates, proteins, fats, vitamins, minerals, fiber and water. For healthy bodies you need to eat the correct quantity and proportion of all these components. You need protein, carbohydrates and fats, for growth, repair and energy. You need vitamins and minerals, albeit in relatively small quantities, so they can perform their vital roles in the thousands of biochemical reactions in your body. Fiber, the broad name given to the foods you eat that your body cannot digest, but that is needed to assist your digestive system.

Complete & Incomplete Proteins

Proteins are molecules of amino acids that are required for cell maintenance and repair, as well as for the regulation of a wide range of bodily functions. Humans need 22 amino acids in order to live. Our bodies can make 14 of the amino acids on their own, but eight of them, called the essential-amino acids, must be acquired from the foods we eat.

Some foods have all the amino acids needed to build other proteins. These are called complete proteins. Nearly every animal food, including dairy products, eggs, meat, poultry and fish are complete proteins because they contain all eight-essential amino acids. Soy is the only plant-based food that has all eight essential-amino acids.

Other plant-based protein sources lack one or more essential amino acids (i.e., amino acids that the body can not either create, or manufacture by modifying other amino acids.) These **incomplete proteins are found in legumes, grains, nuts, and seeds**. Consuming combinations of foods that have incomplete proteins, however, provide the same complete protein end effect as animal protein. **For a complete-protein meal, simply eat any of the incomplete proteins with another but different incomplete protein**, such as eating legumes with grains, or legumes with nuts or seeds, or grains with nuts or seeds. Examples of some healthy plant-protein combinations (that provide complete protein) are pasta and beans, rice and lentils, corn and beans, bean soup with whole-grain bread, split-pea soup with whole-grain bread, peanut butter on whole-grain bread, and tortillas with refried beans. Note that **proteins contain four calories per gram**.

You Need Healthy Carbs

Carbohydrates provide your body with its basic fuel, the energy your cells need to survive. The staple of most diets around the world, carbohydrates provide essential vitamins and minerals, fiber, and numerous beneficial compounds that promote good health.

Simple carbohydrates, such as sugar, taste sweet, and most are digested and enter your bloodstream quickly. When you eat fruit or drink milk, however, the natural sugar comes with vitamins, minerals (as well as fiber when you eat fruit); whereas the simple sugars in candy, for instance, are nothing but nutritionally-empty calories.

Most complex carbohydrates like nearly all grains (wheat, corn, oats, rice) and foods like potatoes, and pasta generally, but not always, are digested more slowly than simple carbohydrates, and take much longer to enter your bloodstream.

When you eat a sweet food, such as a candy bar, or drink a can of soda, your blood glucose level rises rapidly. In response, your pancreas secretes a large amount of insulin to keep your blood glucose levels from rising too high. The large insulin response in turn tends to cause your blood sugar to fall to levels that are too low. As a consequence, about three to five hours after consuming sweets you feel lethargic and hungry. Many people react to this by eating yet another sweet, which can start a rollercoaster ride of surging glucose and then insulin. None of this is experienced after eating most complex carbohydrates, or after a balanced meal, because the digestion and absorption processes are much slower. Note that **carbohydrates contain four calories per gram**.

Fat Facts

Fats are found in vegetable oil, seeds and nuts, meat and fish, and dairy products, as well as in foods like potato chips and french fries (that are cooked in oil), cookies, cake, and so on. There are certain fats you absolutely need to survive (the essential-fatty acids), and others you would do well to drastically limit (saturated fats) or avoid altogether (trans fats). Chemically all fats have the highest calorie density – containing nine calories per gram.

It is becoming increasingly clear that saturated and trans fats, increase the risk for certain diseases while monounsaturated and polyunsaturated fats, lower the risk. Current scientific thinking regarding fat consumption is:

• **Try to limit the total fat you eat** to no more than 30 percent of your caloric intake.

• **Do not consume foods containing partially-hydrogenated vegetable oil** because they are high in trans fats. This includes commercially prepared baked goods, snack foods, and processed foods, including fast foods. To be on the safe-side, assume these food products contain trans fats unless labeled otherwise.

• **Limit saturated fats**, i.e., any fat of animal origin, to 10 percent of your caloric intake. Have meat less often, and when serving meat use lean cuts and trim the fat. Eat fish and poultry (white meat, without the skin) more frequently. Use fat-free or low-fat-milk dairy products in place of whole-milk dairy products.

• When consuming fat, **choose foods containing monounsaturated fats** like olive oil and canola oil, **and foods rich in polyunsaturated omega-6 and omega-3 fatty acids.**

Fat Type	Where found
Saturated	Meat, poultry (especially the skin), dairy products, lard, coconut oil, palm oil, cocoa butter
Trans Fats	Fried foods, margarine, snack foods, commercially-baked cake and cookies, and fast foods
Cholesterol	Egg yokes, dairy products, organ meats, fatty and prime meats, poultry skin, shellfish (particularly
Polyunsaturated (Omega-3)	Mackerel, salmon, sardines, tuna, canola oil, walnuts, flaxseed, wheat germ
Polyunsaturated (Omega-6)	Corn oil, cottonseed oil, safflower oil, sunflower oil, soybean oil
Monounsaturated (Omega-9)	Canola oil, olive oil, safflower oil (hybrid), sunflower oil (hybrid)

Table 2: Fats in Foods

Try to balance your intake essential fatty acids by eating more omega-3 fatty acids, found in walnuts, tofu, certain seeds and oily fish such as salmon, sardines and tuna.

You Need Fiber
Fiber is an important part of a healthy diet. **You need to eat fiber-rich foods to assist your digestive system**. According to the Harvard University School of Public Health, adequate fiber intake reduces the risk of developing various conditions, including heart disease, diabetes, diverticular disease, and constipation. Three fibers that are eaten on a regular basis are cellulose, hemicellulose and pectin. Hemicellulose is found in the hulls of different grains like wheat; e.g., wheat bran is hemicellulose. Cellulose is the structural component of plants, and gives vegetables their familiar shape. Pectin is found most often in fruits, is soluble in water but non-digestible, and is usually referred to as "water-soluble fiber." When you eat fiber, in any of its forms, it simply passes straight through, untouched by but aiding your digestive system. Zero calories absorbed!

Vitamins and Minerals
On the following two pages is a listing of recommended daily allowance for selected vitamins and minerals. Because this is just a "cram course," the best food source for each of the listed vitamins and minerals is not covered in this book.

For much more on nutrition including the basic food groups, good food sources for particular vitamins and minerals, phytonutrients, guidelines for healthy eating, vitamin supplements, advice for seniors, how to estimate the calorie content of a meal, calories in foods, etc. see *Eat Smart - U.S. Edition* another good book published by NoPaperPress.com.

Eat Slowly
One final important point, try to **eat slowly**. This is especially vital if you are on a diet, trying to lose weight. If you are someone who eats fast, who finishes before everyone else at the table, you are not giving yourself a chance to feel full. While everyone else is still eating, you either sit there and pick, or you have seconds, taking in extra calories you could avoid if you would just slow down. To slow down, try eating smaller mouthfuls, try chewing your food more thoroughly, and try talking more at the table.

Vitamin	Men				Women					
	19-30	31-50	51-70	70+	19-30	31-50	51-70	70+	Preg	Lact
A (mcg)	900	900	900	900	700	700	700	700	770	1,300
D (mcg)*	5	5	10	15	5	5	10	15	5	5
E (mcg)	15	15	15	15	15	15	15	15	15	19
K (mcg)*	120	120	120	120	90	90	90	90	90	90
C (mg)	90	90	90	90	75	75	75	75	85	120
B_1 (mg)	1.2	1.2	1.2	1.2	1.1	1.1	1.1	1.1	1.4	1.4
B_2 (mg)	1.3	1.3	1.3	1.3	1.1	1.1	1.1	1.1	1.4	1.6
B_3 (mg)	16	16	16	16	14	14	14	14	18	17
B_5	5	5	5	5	5	5	5	5	6	7
B_6 (mg)	1.3	1.3	1.7	1.7	1.3	1.3	1.5	1.5	1.9	2.0
B_7	30	30	30	30	30	30	30	30	30	35
B_{12}	2.4	2.4	2.4	2.4	2.4	2.4	2.4	2.4	2.6	2.8

Preg = pregnant   Lact = lactating   mcg = micrograms/day   mg = milligram/day
* Vitamins D, K, B_5 and B_7 are "Adequate Intake (AI)" RDAs not established.

Table 3: Recommended Dietary Allowances (RDA) for Selected Vitamins

See next page for RDA for selected minerals.

Mineral	Men				Women					
	19-30	31-50	51-70	70+	19-30	31-50	51-70	70+	Preg	Lact
Calcium (mg)*	1000	1000	1200	1200	1000	1000	1200	1200	1000	1000
Chromium (mcg)*	35	35	30	30	25	25	20	20	30	45
Fluoride (mg)*	4	4	4	4	3	3	3	3	3	3
Iodine (mcg)	150	150	150	150	150	150	150	150	220	290
Iron (mg)	8	8	8	8	18	18	8	8	27	9
Magnesium (mg)	400	420	420	420	310	320	320	320	355	315
Manganese (mg)*	2.3	2.3	2.3	2.3	1.8	1.8	1.8	1.8	2.0	2.6
Molybdenum	45	45	45	45	45	45	45	45	50	50
Phosphorus (mg)	700	700	700	700	700	700	700	700	700	700
Potassium (mg)	4700	4700	4700	4700	4700	4700	4700	4700	4700	5100
Selenium (mcg)	55	55	55	55	55	55	55	55	60	70
Zinc (mg)	11	11	11	11	8	8	8	8	8	8

Preg = pregnant   Lact = lactating   mcg = micrograms/day   mg = milligrams/day
* Calcium, chromium, fluoride & manganese are "Adequate Intake (AI)."

Table 4. Recommended Dietary Allowances (RDA) for Selected Minerals

4. Exercise Basics

There are two ways to become more physically active: 1) Increase the physical activity in your daily life; and 2) Start on a regular exercise program. Better still would be a combination of both. Here are some ways you can increase physical activity during daily living:

- Change your attitude toward the occasional "bothersome" physical tasks that you encounter in daily living. Consider anytime you have to lift, bend, reach, walk as an opportunity to burn additional calories and as an extension of your formal workout.

- Look for opportunities to walk, such as walking up stairs (two at a time if you can) rather than using an elevator, walking to a local store rather than driving, walking the course if you play golf, and mowing your lawn. At work stand up and stretch at least every two hours, read standing up, etc.

- Engage in leisure activities such as dancing, bowling and gardening as often as you can. They can be enjoyable and provide added exercise.

Each of these daily activities taken alone may not seem like much, but done most days for many years they can add up to a substantial number of extra calories burned.

Select the Right Exercise

Selecting the right fitness exercise is the key to a successful regular conditioning program. You should try to pick an activity (or activities) you will enjoy. Factors to consider in choosing your activity are: your medical condition, your age, your fitness level, your exercise goals, your daily and overall schedule, do you prefer to exercise outdoors or indoors, exercise alone or with others, and how much money you are prepared to spend. You may decide to concentrate on one activity such as squash, or you may choose to walk briskly some days and lift weights on other days. Incidentally, three to five days of a vigorous aerobic exercise plus two days of either strength or flexibility exercises per week is a good combination. Whatever you settle on make sure it is an activity (or activities) that can be done regularly and that you enjoy.

Aerobic Exercise: How Hard?

The central part of your exercise program should be an aerobic (or cardio) exercise done regularly. Additional stretching and strengthening exercises should be included as time allows – but never to the exclusion of the aerobic portion of your program.

An aerobic exercise program should be vigorous enough to condition your cardiovascular system but not so strenuous as to exceed safe limits. Some experts define safe as an exercise pace that is "comfortable." What they mean is that if, for instance, you are jogging or walking briskly you should be able to converse comfortably with a partner and that you should be breathing and feeling normally within ten minutes after you stop exercising. If not, you are exercising too vigorously. Other signs that you are pushing too hard include difficulty breathing, feeling faint, or feeling weak – during or after exercising. If you experience any of these symptoms, you are exercising too intensely and you should cut back.

Activity	Weight (lbs.)								
	120	140	160	180	200	220	240	260	280
Aerobics (dance)	491	573	655	736	818	900	982	1064	1145
Basketball	382	445	509	573	636	700	764	827	891
Bicycling (13 mph)	435	508	580	653	725	798	870	943	1015
Cycling (stationary)	382	445	509	573	636	700	764	827	891
Calisthenics	341	398	455	511	568	625	682	739	795
Dancing (ballroom)	250	292	333	375	417	458	500	542	583
Golf (pulling cart)	270	315	360	405	450	495	540	585	630
Golf (riding cart)	190	222	253	285	317	348	380	412	443
Hiking	320	373	427	480	533	587	640	693	747
Hockey (ice/field)	430	502	573	645	717	788	860	932	1003
Jogging 8 min/mile	680	793	907	1020	1133	1247	1360	1473	1587
Mowing lawn	299	349	399	449	499	549	599	649	699
Rowing (moderate)	380	443	507	570	633	697	760	823	887

Table 5 continues on the following page.

Sitting (watch TV)	70	82	93	105	117	128	140	152	163
Skating	380	443	507	570	633	697	760	823	887
Skiing (X country)	435	508	580	653	725	798	870	943	1015
Skiing (downhill)	330	385	440	495	550	605	660	715	770
Skipping rope	457	533	609	686	762	838	914	990	1067
Soccer	410	479	547	615	684	752	820	889	957
Swimming laps	440	513	587	660	733	807	880	953	1027
Tennis (singles)	320	373	427	480	533	587	640	693	747
Tennis (doubles)	243	283	324	364	405	445	485	526	566
Walking (3mph)	194	227	259	291	324	356	388	421	453
Walking (3.5 mph)	238	277	317	357	396	436	476	515	555
Walking (4 mph)	302	353	403	453	504	554	604	655	705

Table 5 Caloric Cost (per hour) for Various Activities

If your goal is to burn calories to control your weight and to improve your general health and fitness, walking is a wonderful exercise. Walking does have a downside. Because it is a relatively low-intensity exercise, to get a good workout you have to spend more time walking compared to many other high-intensity exercises.

Get a Pedometer - Count Steps
Sedentary people only take about 2000 to 3000 steps a day. For the average person with a stride equal to about 2.5 feet (0.75 m), 2,100 steps amounts to walking about one mile (1.6 km).

A Harvard University study has shown that 6000 steps a day correlate with lower death rates in men, and that 8000 to 10,000 step per day promote weight loss. And these health and weight management benefits don't oblige you to walk continuously until you accrue the required number of steps. Rather, all steps throughout the day to wherever and whenever count toward your daily total.

Strength-Building Programs
As good as aerobic exercises are, they contribute little to building upper-body strength. If you are a beginner interested in strength training it's

probably worthwhile to start by joining a health club, where you can get professional instruction on the proper use of exercise equipment, from dumbbells to rowing machines, and where you can compare different exercise routines and develop a personalized fitness program.

Of all the many strength-building options, I personally prefer free weights (actually dumbbells) because they can be used at home. Working out at home has some significant advantages. First, your workout takes less time because you don't have to drive back and forth to a health club; second, you have the flexibility of dividing your workout into small time segments to fit your day, whenever you have time, such as when the baby is napping, and of course working out at home is certainly less expensive.

You can workout in a bedroom, basement, garage, attic – anywhere you have extra space. A set of variable (adjustable) weight dumbbells and a small weight bench don't take up much room and are all you need for a home-based gym. Choose dumbbell exercises that comprise a total-body workout, that are suitable for beginners, and that involve all the major muscle groups. Bear in mind, **knowledge and the discipline to work out regularly are far more important than fancy equipment.**

Risks and Possible Problems
Certain situations may occur that indicate you may be doing too much, exercising too hard. For example, regardless of your pulse rate you should never be left completely breathless by your aerobic exercise. A good rule to remember is: **You are exercising too hard if you cannot carry on a conversation while you are jogging, cycling, etc**. A feeling of having worked hard is fine, sweating is good, but not a feeling of undo fatigue.

Perhaps the most frequent problems faced by exercisers are injuries of the joints and muscles: sprains and strains, knee pain, elbow pain, back pain, neck pain, shin splints and stress fractures. Most happen when you exercise too hard.

Potentially serious problems are signaled if you experience any of the following symptoms during or after exercise. The symptoms include but are not limited to any abnormal heart action, such as an irregular heart rhythm, pain or pressure in the middle of your chest, pain in an arm or your neck, dizziness, fainting or lightheadedness, severe exhaustion, sudden loss of coordination, or confusion. If any of these symptoms are experienced, stop exercising immediately and get medical help.

Avoiding Injury

My good friend and frequent workout buddy, A.C. Kanaar, M.D., specialized in rehabilitation medicine but he also preached what he called "preventive medicine," that is avoiding injury by practicing a common-sense approach to exercise:

- Have a medical checkup and then set realistic fitness goals.
- Build up your exercise intensity gradually over many weeks, months.
- After you eat a meal, wait about two hours before exercising.
- Buy good equipment suitable for your exercise routine.
- Use safety and protective equipment when appropriate, such as helmet when you bicycle, and goggles when you play handball, squash or racquetball.
- Don't exercise on very hot day or very cold days.
- If you insist on working out in very hot or cold weather, always let someone know when and where you will be exercising and when you are planning to return.
- If you are new to a gym or health club, attend an orientation session before you use any unfamiliar exercise equipment. Otherwise, read the operating instructions carefully, and ask someone qualified for help.
- For aerobic activities, warm up slowly and cool down slowly after you exercise.
- Do not increase the difficulty of any activity (e.g., your walking or jogging distance, the amount of weight you lift) by more than 10 percent per week.
- Jog on softer surfaces such as a level grass field, a dirt path, or a running track.
- After exercising wait 30 minutes before eating.
- As a final point, if you experience some early warning pain stop exercising.

Remember it doesn't matter exactly what exercises you choose, what equipment you use, or what facility you use. These are secondary factors. What matters most is that you exercise consistently.

To improve muscle tone and overall fitness, feel good and stay healthy, you should exercise at least five days per week, day after day, week after week, year after year – for as long as you are physically able. Remember the key words: consistent, determined, steady, persistent, dogged, unswerving, gritty, single-minded. Consistent!

For much more on exercise I recommend *Exercise **Smart - U.S. Edition*** another excellent book again published by NoPaperPress.

5. About Your Weight

Why are you overweight? Once you accept the fact that your weight is governed by the conservation of energy, the answer is simple enough. You are overweight because you consume more calories than you expend. Overeating or inactivity, or a combination of both, are the culprits. But they are the cause of your overweight, not the reason for it.

The question might more properly be: Why do you eat more than you should? The popular notion that most people are overweight or obese because of a defect in their metabolism is just not supported by scientific evidence. In fact, being overweight or obese most often can be attributed to how we adapt to our 21st century environment and to our heredity. More specifically, the major causes of obesity and overweight are as follows:

- **Environmental**: We live in a society where food is abundant and where strenuous physical activity is, for most people, a thing of the past. In other words, we eat too much and do too little. This is by far the most important factor.

- **Genetic**: Everyone starts life with a different body type. Researchers agree there is a relationship between the body type we inherit and the likelihood and ease with which we become overweight. Three basic body types are illustrated in the figure on the next page. The active ectomorph, with a typically long, narrow body and light appetite will find it difficult indeed to gain weight or to become overweight. On the other extreme, the more sedentary endomorph with a hearty appetite faces a life-long struggle against obesity. Depending on their appetite and how active they are, even muscular mesomorphs often gain unwanted weight as they age. Because everyone has some features of each body type, we are all born with different weight gaining tendencies.

- **Psychological**: There are a great many people who overeat and become overweight in response to tension, frustration, or other psychological issues.

- **Developmental**: Early forced feeding often leads to childhood-onset obesity. Overeating then becomes habitual and an excessive number of fat cells are formed early on that are difficult to shed later in life.

- **Metabolic and Regulatory**: Sometimes overeating is caused by a damaged hypothalamus or an incorrect interpretation of the hunger/satiety signal. Though relatively rare, a defect in the thyroid or pituitary gland can also cause a change in metabolic rate. All can result in overweight. I am going to assume that you have consulted with your physician and have no physiological disorder (glandular, digestive, etc.) that would prevent you from losing weight. Very few people are overweight because of this sort of ailment.

The fact is that although you may never understand the underlying cause for your being overweight, you still can do something about it. You can still lose weight successfully by understanding and applying the basics of sound diet theory.

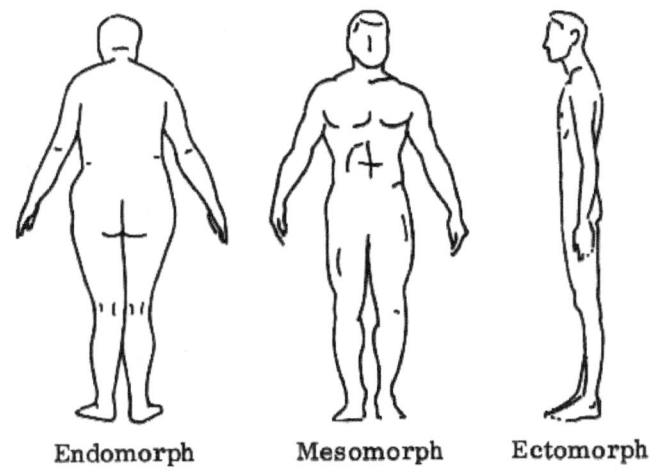

    Endomorph   Mesomorph   Ectomorph

Human Body Types

What You Should Weigh

Body Weight Mass Index, or BMI is currently the method used by physicians and researchers to assess a person's weight. To utilize the common place BMI chart, one enters the chart with their height and weight and determines their BMI. Then another chart is used to convert the BMI into a weight profile.

I devised a more convenient way, that is to use a New BMI-Based Weight vs. Height Chart shown in Table 6, (on the next page) where the underweight category corresponds to BMI = 18.5 or less, normal weight is for BMI = 18.6 to 24.9, overweight is for BMI = 25.0 to 29.9, obese is for BMI = 30.0 to 39.9 and extremely obese is for BMI = 40 or more. Readers should strive to get their BMI into the normal category, or 18.6 to 24.9. As an example, let's consider data from President Trump's 2018 physical exam. The president's physician determined that the president is 6' 3" and 239 lbs. Overweight. But from Table 6, one can see that if the president weighed just one pound more, or 240 lbs, he would be considered obese.

Height	Underweight (lbs)	Normal Weight (lbs)	Overweight (lbs)	Obese (lbs)	Extremely Obese (lbs)
5' 0"	95 or less	96 – 127	128 – 152	153 – 204	≥ 205
5' 1"	98 or less	99 – 131	132 – 158	159 – 211	≥ 212
5' 2"	101 or less	102 – 135	136 – 163	164 – 218	≥ 219
5' 3"	104 or less	105 – 140	141 – 169	170 – 225	≥ 226
5' 4"	108 or less	109 – 144	145 – 173	174 – 232	≥ 233
5' 5"	111 or less	112 – 149	150 – 180	181 – 239	≥ 240
5' 6"	115 or less	116 – 154	155 – 185	186 – 247	≥ 248
5' 7"	118 or less	119 – 159	160 – 191	192 – 254	≥ 255
5' 8"	122 or less	123 – 163	164 – 196	197 – 262	≥ 263
5' 9"	125 or less	126 – 168	169 – 202	203 – 270	≥ 271
5' 10"	129 or less	130 – 173	174 – 206	207 – 278	≥ 279
5' 11"	133 or less	134 – 178	179 – 214	215 – 286	≥ 287
6' 0"	136 or less	137 – 183	184 – 220	221 – 294	≥ 295
6' 1"	140 or less	141 – 188	189 – 227	228 – 302	≥ 303
6' 2"	144 or less	145 – 194	195 – 232	233 – 310	≥ 311
6' 3"	148 or less	149 – 199	200 – 239	240 – 319	≥ 320
6' 4"	152 or less	153 – 204	205 – 245	246 – 328	≥ 329
6' 5"	156 or less	157 – 210	211 – 252	253 – 336	≥ 337

Table 6: New BMI-Based Weight vs. Height

Body Fat Percentage

Many health care professionals contend that overweight or obesity does not depend on body weight but on the amount of body fat a person carries compared to their total body weight.

Body fat exists in two storage sites. The first storage depot, consists of the intestines, muscles, and the lipid-rich tissues throughout the central nervous system. This is referred to as Essential Fat and is required, or essential to maintain health. In females, essential fat also includes sex-specific or sex-characteristic fat. The average woman requires approximately 10% essential fat, and the average man about 3%. The higher percentage of essential fat in females includes about 7% of sex-specific fat, believed to be important for child-bearing and other hormone-related functions.

This is an important topic but is beyond the scope of this book. For more information, including the following new unique tables: Body Fat Percentage, Maximum Waist Size, Optimum Waist Size, Waist to Hip Ratio, see *Professional Weight Control - U.S. Edition* an eBook also published by NoPaperPress.com.

6. Weight Loss

In the short term only, the energy value of weight change is approximately 3500 Calories for one pound of weight lost or gained. But for longer duration diets with more weight loss, this rule does not apply. In most practical diet situations, the Weight Loss Prediction model I developed, or the Weight Loss Prediction Tables must be used.

Diet Options

Once you have utilized **Table 1** (on page 17) to settle on your Activity Level, you are ready to use the Weight Loss Prediction tables, to determine your diet calorie options. Weight Loss Prediction Tables are located in **Appendix A for Men** (on page 52) and in **Appendix B for Women**, (on page 125) and are organized by gender, age, height, weight and activity level. Use of the tables is best illustrated by an example.

WEIGHT LOSS PREDICTION FOR WOMEN Ages: 18 to 35 yrs.

Height: 4' 11" to 5' 5"   Activity Level 1

Weight Loss	Diet Calories	Present Weight (lbs.)							
		110	120	130	140	160	180	200	220
5	900	19	17	16	15		11	10	9
5	1200	28	24	21	19		14	12	11
5	1500	49	39	32	28		18	15	13
5	1800	210	99	66	49		25	20	17
10	900	40	36	33	30		23	21	19
10	1200	58	50	44	40		29	25	23
10	1500	106	82	68	58		37	32	28
10	1800		234	145	106		52	42	35
15	900		55	51	46		36	32	29
15	1200		78	69	62		44	39	35
15	1500		132	107	91		57	49	42
15	1800			245	172		81	65	55
20	900			76	69	63	55	48	44	40
20	1200			108	95		70	60	53	47
20	1500			188	151		96	78	66	58
20	1800			380	252		154	113	89	74
30	900			109	100	86	75	67	61
30	1200			153	135	110	94	82	73
30	1500			257	209	155	124	104	90

Table 7: Portion of Table B.1 (Illustrates Example 1)

Example 1: A 28-year-old woman, who is 5' 3" and 160 pounds, is a computer programmer, and spends most of her free time watching TV. How long will it take her to lose 20 pounds?

Considering her job and leisure-time pursuits, from Table 1, (on page 17) she decides she is Activity Level 1. Next she consults Appendix B (on page 89) and finds the Weight Loss Prediction table that applies to her is Table B.1, (on page 90) labeled "Weight Loss Prediction: Women 18 to 35 yrs, 4' 11" to 5' 5", Activity Level 1." Table 7, above, shows a portion of Table B.1.

To use the portion of Table B.1 shown above, our dieter would scan the far left of the table and locate her desired weight loss of 20 pounds. There she finds four different diet options of 900, 1200, 1500 and 1800 Calories. From this point, she runs a finger horizontally (to the right) until it intersects the vertical column headed by her present weight of 160 pounds. The four highlighted numbers in the box are the time in days to lose 20 pounds, depending on the diet calories consumed. Specifically, to lose 20 pounds our fictional female's diet calorie options are:

- 900 Calories per day for 55 days.
- 1200 Calories per day for 70 days.
- 1500 Calories per day for 96 days.
- 1800 Calories per day for 154 days.

Which alternative should she choose? Many health-care professionals recommend a gradual weight loss of one to two pounds per week. The reason for the relatively slow weight loss is that you want to be on the diet long enough to understand and learn how much to eat, and how to eat properly. In this case, at two pounds per week her diet should last 10 weeks or 70 days, and at one pound per week her diet should take 20 weeks or 140 days.

To comply with accepted weight loss guidelines, therefore, she should choose a diet calorie level that will result in her losing the 20 pounds over a 70 to 140 day period – pointing to the 1200 or 1500-Calorie options. In the end, it comes down to her deciding between the shorter term 1200-Calorie diet or a longer duration somewhat higher 1500-Calorie option.

Better still would be for this woman to increase her activity level by taking a brisk three-mile walk everyday, and qualifying for Activity Level 2, the moderately active category (**Table B.2** on page 91) which would result in the following shorter-duration diet options:

- 900 Calories per day for 47 days.
- 1200 Calories per day for 57 days.
- 1500 Calories per day for 74 days.
- 1800 Calories per day for 104 days.

Hence, by increasing her activity level, she could decrease the time to lose the 20 pounds by 14 to 32 percent – depending on the diet-calorie level she chooses.

Suppose Your Weight Isn't In Table?
Suppose the woman in Example 1 weighed 190 pounds and wanted to lose 30 pounds on a 1200-Calorie Diet. But 190 pounds is not listed in Table B.1. on page 90. No problem. By noting that the time required to lose 30 pounds when weighing 190 pounds would be half-way between the times shown in the table for 180 and 200 pounds, she would proceed as follows. First, from Table B.1, she would find that that on a 1200-Calorie diet, at 180 pounds it would take her 94 days to lose 30 pounds, and at 200 pounds it would take 82 days. The time on a 1200-Calorie diet at 190 pounds would be in the middle of these two, or 88 days. This estimating technique is called interpolation and should be used whenever you can't find your exact weight in one of the tables. If math was never your strong suit, don't give up! Get a friend to help. The important part – the doing – comes after the calculations. That's where you come in.

The Physiology of Weight Loss
Weight lost during periods of negative energy balance is of variable composition. Fat, water, and protein are lost at different rates and at different stages of a reducing diet. The amount of water in humans also varies from day to day. Over reasonable period of time, however, the amount of water entering the body will equal the amount leaving. And the water balance of the body is then said to be in equilibrium.

A considerable loss of water usually occurs at the start of a diet. Because a pint of water weighs about one pound, this initial water loss will appear as a weight loss. But the weight loss is not "real," because no body tissue has been lost. (From this point on, when reference is made to "real" weight loss, what is meant is that weight loss which will not be regained, once the body's water balance is restored.)

Many theories have been proposed to explain this phenomenon but none have been confirmed scientifically. Because of changes in body hydration, you will usually notice higher weight loss during the first week or two on a diet than the Weight Loss Prediction Tables forecast. By the following week, however, the water balance of the body will readjust and your weight loss will more closely approach the values in the Weight Loss Prediction Tables. The tables predict "real" weight loss. In addition, realize that the weight of a normal person fluctuates two to three pounds daily. Your weight is lowest before breakfast and highest in the evening before retiring. So to determine your weight loss, always weigh yourself at the same time of day.

In women, another cause of weight fluctuation is water retention just prior to their menstrual period. This is not uncommon and may appear to be a time when weight is not lost. Again, by the next week, the water balance of the body will readjust and your weight loss will more closely approach the values in the Weight Loss Prediction Tables.

Weight Loss Principles
Once the parameters involved in weight loss are related in a mathematical equation, it is possible to state some principles. (It is also possible to deduce the following truisms by examining the Weight Loss Prediction tables.)

• Given two people the same age, gender and activity level, and on the same reducing diet, **the heavier person will lose weight faster than the thinner person**. For instance, according to **Table A.1** on page 53, on 1500 Calories, it would take a 25-year old, 5'-4", 140-pound male (Activity Level 1) 48 days to lose 10 pounds; whereas the same table indicates a 240-pound male on 1500 Calories would only take 22 days to lose 10 pounds – less than half the time!

• Given two people the same age, gender and activity level, and on the same reducing diet (i.e., consuming the same number of calories), the taller person will lose weight at a slightly faster rate.

- Given a male and female, the same age, weight, activity level and on the same reducing diet, **the man will lose weight faster than the woman**. This happens because women have lower basal metabolic rates than men and therefore must eat less than a man to lose the same amount of weight.

- Given two individuals, the same gender, weight and activity level, **the younger person will lose weight much faster than the older person.** The lesson is if you are overweight start on a weight loss diet now because it will only become **more difficult to lose weight as you get older.**

- It follows that if your **caloric intake is constant over the years you will slowly gain weight as you age.** This is because your basal metabolic rate decreases as you advance in age, and most people tend not to be as active as they get older.

Selecting a Weight Loss Diet
As mentioned previously, this book does not actually contain a diet. But there are sample 1200 and 1500 Calorie **nutritionally balanced diets** (see **Chapter 8,** starting on page 44), all with sample no-cooking and cooking daily meal plans complete with sample recipes.

The sample diets give you an idea of how much food you can eat at a given calorie level. Of course, on a 900 Calorie diet you would be eating 300 Calories less than on the 1200 Calorie diet, and on an 1800 Calorie diet you would have 300 Calories more to eat than on a 1500 Calorie diet.

Incidentally, a 900 Calorie diet is usually not recommended. This is because it is difficult to obtain all the nutrients you need on 900 Calories, and it is also difficult to stay on a very low calorie diet over the long term.

Use the weight loss prediction tables in conjunction with the activity level table, and then the sample 1200 and 1500 Calorie weight loss daily meal plans to help you select the diet calorie level that is best for you. Only 1200 and 1500 meal plans are shown here, but be aware that 900 and 1800 Calorie plans are also available in some NoPaperPress eBooks.

Once you decide on your diet calorie level, you can navigate to NoPaperPress.com for complete 7-Day, 30-Day, 60-Day, 90-Day and 100-Day diets - both cooking and no-cooking. Incidentally, **no-cooking diet books are unique to NoPaperPress**.

7. Weight Maintenance

Most people can lose weight on almost any diet, but the crucial issue is whether the weight loss can be maintained. The real challenge is not losing weight but keeping it off! Few, if any, of the popular weight control programs have been successful at maintaining weight over the long term. There are two key concerns with respect to weight maintenance:

1. **Preventing people from gaining weight as they age**.

2. **Preventing the regaining of lost weight, i.e., helping people keep off weight they've lost**.

In fact both of these vexing issues can be approached and solved using virtually the same weight control techniques. First you need to understand why you gain or regain weight.

Why You Gain Weight With Age

A study, published in a 2005 issue of the Annals of Internal Medicine, that followed 4000 adults for three decades suggests that in the long term, 90 percent of men and 70 percent of women will become overweight (with a BMI ≥ 25). Interestingly, half of the men and women in the study, who had made it well into adulthood without a weight problem, ultimately also became overweight and a third became obese (BMI ≥ 30).

Why does this happen? When you reach your mid to late twenties, you slowly start to lose muscle and add fat as part of the natural aging process. As you age your muscle mass slowly deteriorates and is replaced by fat. But muscle is active tissue and requires lots of energy (calories) for growth and repair; whereas, fat is basically inactive and uses very few calories to exist. So as you age and you lose muscle mass your metabolism gradually slows.

In fact your metabolism decreases about 10 percent every decade. If you are like the average adult, at some point, because of your slowing metabolism, you could start to gain 1½ to 2 pounds every year. To offset this, you need to cut back on calories, or increase your physical activity, or both. Otherwise the excess calories will add up and so will your weight! The point being that you can never become complacent. **You must**

continually watch your weight because we are all at risk of becoming overweight.

Why You Gain Weight After a Diet
After any diet, your lower body weight requires fewer calories to function. In other words, your lower body weight results in a slower overall metabolism. Within five years, most dieters regain every pound they have lost. Why? In most cases it's because after losing weight most people eventually revert to their pre-diet eating and exercising habits, and this inevitably leads to their regaining the weight they lost – and often more. The fact is **the less you weigh, the less you need to eat to maintain your lower weight**.

Without some lifestyle modifications, if you are like the average adult you will regain every pound you have lost. It's a fact that 95 percent of dieters, that's 95 out of 100 people, regain all the weight they lost and often more!

People Who Regained Lost Weight
A study published in the American Journal of Preventive Medicine, surveyed about 1300 adults from the 1999 to 2002 who were overweight or obese and had lost at least 10 percent of their maximum weight. The study authors found some common characteristics associated with those who regained lost weight:

- They spent four hours or more per day in front of a TV set or computer.
- They lost a lot of weight (at least 20% of their max. weight) in a short time.
- They started regaining lost weight soon after they stopped dieting.

Most of the above make sense. Too much TV or computer time usually means these people were undoubtedly sedentary and less likely to get lots of exercise.

Losing weight too fast, either by fad or extreme dieting, can leave people feeling deprived and often ends up triggering binges that go on until the lost weight is regained.

It takes time to establish a new lifestyle that supports weight maintenance.

People who have lost weight and then quickly gained it back, may not have had the time to acquire all the skills needed to maintain their lower weight.

People Who Maintained Lost Weight
The National Weight Control Registry studied people who had lost at least 30 pounds and kept it off for more than a year. What they found was that **although people lost weight differently, they kept it off similarly**. Here are some common traits of the successful maintainers:

- Most maintainers ate a low-fat diet - but not a hugely restrictive one.
- All successful maintainers monitor their portion sizes.
- Nearly four in five eat breakfast every day.
- Most are physically active, with walking their most common activity.
- They walk for nearly an hour every day.
- They weighed themselves once a week.
- These people probably were not spending four plus hours watching TV.
- They found pleasure in their healthier lifestyle and freedom from constant dieting.

Select Correct Weight Maintenance Table
The Weight Maintenance Calorie tables display how many the calories you can eat without gaining or losing weight. Or put another way how many calories you can consume and not regain your lost weight.

First, you need to select the Weight Maintenance Table that's right for you. The tables are organized by gender, age, height, weight and activity level. In this book you will find an updated set of 15 Weight Maintenance Calorie tables in **Appendix C for men** on page 114 and in **Appendix D for women** on page 124.

How to Use the Weight Maintenance Tables
Use of the Weight Maintenance Tables is best illustrated by the following example.

Example 2:   Consider a 53-year-old, 5'-8", woman, relatively inactive (Activity Level 1), who weighed 200 pounds at the start of her reducing diet. After losing 50 pounds, she weighed 150 pounds. Determine her weight maintenance calories before and after she lost weight.

From **Table D.4** on page 128 she finds that before she started her diet, when she weighed 200 pounds, her weight maintenance level was 2741 Calories, meaning she must have been eating about 2741 Calories of food per day.

After her diet, the same table shows that in order to maintain her lower weight of 150 pounds she

must restrict her food intake in the future to 2297 Calories per day. On average, then, to neither gain nor lose weight at 150 pounds she must eat about 2741 − 2297 = 444 Calories per day less than she ate when she weighed 200 pounds.

This person could help her cause by engaging in some form of exercise every day. For example, if she walked 45 minutes every day at moderate 3.5 mph pace (covering a distance of slightly more than 2½ miles), she could eat an additional 160 Calories per day without gaining weight.

Weight Maintenance is a Life-Long Struggle
A trim 43 year-old nutritionist laughs when people say, "Oh, you're so lucky to be naturally thin." Her reply, "Give me break. I workout and do you think I eat everything I want?"

Staying lean requires constant vigilance. In weight maintenance, it is the number of calories you eat over the long term that is important. As an illustration, the weight maintenance value of 2297 Calories per day for the 53-year-old woman in Example 2 amounts to about 838,000 Calories in a single year. Now realize that an annual error of only two percent of this total (that is roughly 16800 Calories per year, or 46 Calories per day) would result in a weight gain of (16800 Calories / 3500 Calories per lb = 4.8 lbs) almost five pounds in one year, and the importance of knowing and adhering to your personal weight maintenance calorie value becomes apparent. In brief, **to control your weight it is the number of calories eaten over the long term that matters**.

Obviously, it would be impossible for the woman in Example 2 to eat exactly 2297 Calories day after day. Errors are inevitable and experience has shown that when people err they do so on the high side. They consume more calories than their maintenance value, rarely less. To allow for occasional overeating or days when don't have time to exercise, it is recommended that you plan to eat about seven percent below the calorie values in the weight maintenance tables. For the female in Example 2, that would mean about 2140 Calories per day rather than the 2297 Calories shown in the weight maintenance calorie table – leaving her room for an occasional calorie splurge, or a missed exercise session.

Get Off the Diet Roller Coaster
For most people, a shape-up program consists of getting on the latest diet bandwagon. But short-term diets are temporary and rarely work. It makes no sense to go on a diet for a few months, only to regain the weight. Losing weight is comparatively easy; the challenging part is keeping it off. Instead of short-term fixes, you should focus on developing better eating and exercise habits – that you can stay with over the long haul. Instead of going on and off diets, you should change our approach and make exercise and good nutrition a way of life.

Get off the diet roller coaster once and for all by developing habits that you will be able to maintain for the rest of your life. It may take a little more discipline, patience and hard work this way, but it the end it will all be worth it. To lose weight permanently, you must make a commitment to a healthier way of life. So get started.

8. Sample Weight Loss & Maintenance Diets

In this chapter you will be introduced to 1200 and 1500 Calorie sample weight loss diets and a 2500 Calorie weight maintenance meal plan. The purpose of these sample diets is to help you appreciate how much food you can eat at these calorie levels.

Weight Loss: 1200 and 1500 Calorie diets are most often recommended by health care professionals. Use the 1200 and 1500 Calorie sample daily menus to understand how much food you can eat at these calorie levels

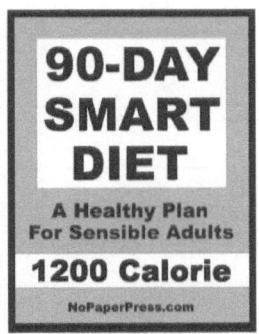
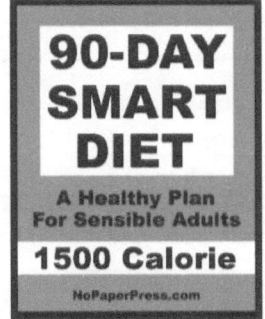
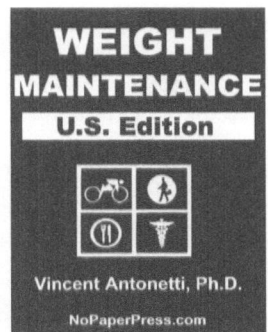

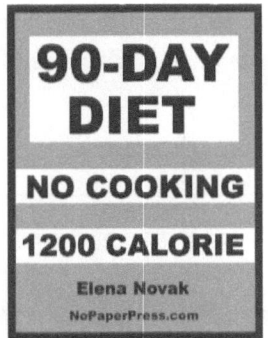
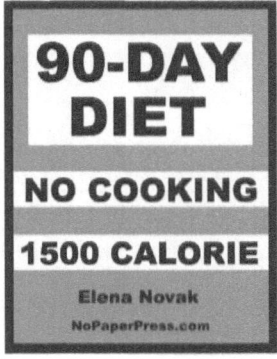

Weight Maintenance: After using the Weight Maintenance tables to determine the appropriate calorie level for your new lower weight, add or subtract calories from the sample 2500 Calorie weight maintenance meal plan to understand how much food you can eat without regaining weight.

The following 1200 and 1500 Calorie diets and the 2500 Calorie weight maintenance plan are from the preceding NoPaperPress eBooks with permission.

Table 8. Sample 1200 Calorie Daily Meal Plan

BREAKFAST	Calories	Totals
Orange juice (½ cup)	50	
Wheaties (¾ cup) + ½ cup skim milk + ½ banana	190	
Whole-grain toast (1 slice)	70	
Coffee	10	320 Cal
SNACK		
Fresh fruit in season (apple, pear, etc)	70	
Coffee or tea	10	80 Cal
LUNCH		
Microwaveable Soup #10 (See Appendix B)	110	
Turkey breast (1 oz) on 1 slice rye bread (½	105	
Lettuce & tomato slices	20	
Hot or iced tea	10	245 Cal
SNACK		
Coffee or tea	10	10 Cal
DINNER		
Baked Herb-Crusted Cod (Day 2 Recipe)	230	
Spinach (½ cup) steamed with garlic & drizzled	100	
Asparagus (8 spear cooked & drained)	25	
Baked potato (medium size) (No Butter!)	100	
Whole-grain bread (1 slice)	70	
Water with lemon wedge	10	535 Cal
SNACK		
Coffee or tea	10	10 Cal
		1200 Cal

Table from NoPaperPress eBook: *90-Day Smart Diet - 1200 Calorie* with permission.

Day 2 - Recipe

<u>Baked Herb-Crusted Cod</u>

4 cod fish fillets (4 to 5 ounces each)
2 tablespoons flour
2 tablespoons cornmeal
2 tablespoons minced fresh herbs
2 teaspoons lemon juice

Sprinkle cod with lemon juice. Mix flour, cornmeal and herbs and dust the cod with the cornmeal-herb mixture. Bake in oven at 375 °F for 10 minutes. Add salt and black pepper to taste.

<u>Serves 4</u>. One serving is about 230 Calories (for cod only).

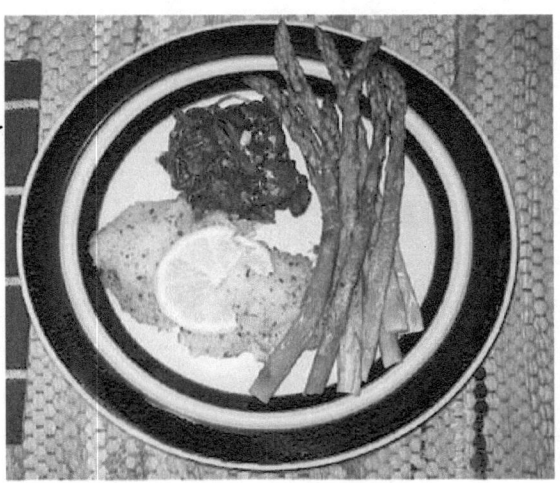

<u>Diet Tip of the Day:</u> When you're on a diet, eating in a restaurant can be a challenge, because most restaurant portions are huge, and can easily total more than 1,000 Calories. So, in a restaurant decide how much to eat – and take the remainder home. A good general rule of thumb is to **eat half and bring the rest home**.

Recipe from NoPaperPress eBook: *90-Day Smart Diet - 1200 Calorie* with permission.

Table 9: Sample 1500 Calorie Daily Meal Plan

BREAKFAST	Calories	Totals
Grapefruit (½)	75	
Cheerios (1 cup) + ½ cup skim milk + about 15	190	
Coffee	10	275 Cal
SNACK		
Handful unsalted mixed nuts	100	
Coffee or tea	10	110 Cal
LUNCH		
Cottage cheese (1 cup low fat)	180	
Large tossed salad with 1½ Tbsp low-cal dressing	70	
Small whole-grain roll	80	
Hot or iced tea	10	340 Cal
SNACK		
Fresh fruit in season (peach, plum, etc)	70	
Coffee or tea	10	80 Cal
DINNER		
Grilled swordfish (Day 18 Recipe)	250	
Grilled potatoes (See Day 18 Recipe)	100	
Grilled cherry tomatoes (See Day 18 Recipe)	45	
Spinach (½ cup) steamed with garlic & drizzled	50	
Whole-grain bread (1 slice)	70	
Water with lemon wedge	10	525 Cal
SNACK		
Two small cookies	160	
Coffee or tea	10	170 Cal
		1500 Cal

Table from NoPaperPress eBook: *90-Day Smart Diet - 1500 Calorie* with permission.

Day 18 - Recipe

Grilled Swordfish

1¼ pounds swordfish
1 bottle citrus-herb marinade
¾ pint cherry tomatoes (about 20), halved
4 medium potatoes
2 cups fresh spinach
1 teaspoon rosemary & juice of ¼ lemon
2 teaspoon extra-virgin olive oil, divided

- Steam spinach with garlic and drizzle with about 1 teaspoon extra-virgin olive oil.
- Cut potatoes in medium-size pieces and sprinkle with lemon juice, add rosemary, salt and black pepper. Place potatoes on grill for about 10 minutes, turning occasionally.
- Toss cherry tomatoes in remaining extra-virgin olive oil. Add fresh oregano, salt and black pepper. Place on heavy-duty aluminum foil, seal and grill for about 3 minutes.
- Marinade swordfish in citrus-herb vinaigrette. Grill on hot fire for about 5 minutes on one side and 3 minutes on the other, or until done as desired.

Serves 4. One plate of grilled swordfish (250 Calories) with potatoes (100 Calories), cherry tomatoes (45 Calories) and steamed spinach (50 Calories) totals 445 Calories.

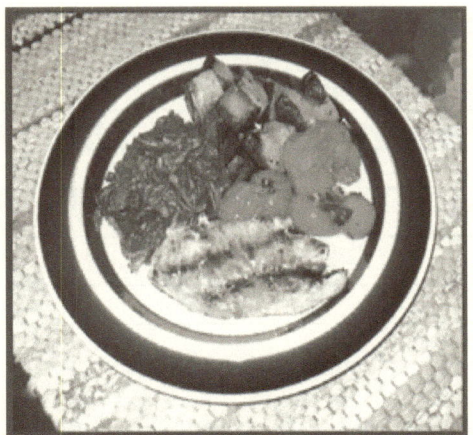

Recipe from NoPaperPress eBook: *90-Day Smart Diet - 1500 Calorie* with permission.

Table 10: Sample 1500 Calorie No-Cooking Daily Meal Plan

BREAKFAST	Calories	Totals
Fresh sliced orange	75	
Wheaties (¾ cup) + ½ cup skim milk + ½ banana	190	
Whole-grain toast (1 slice)	70	
Coffee	10	345 Cal
SNACK		
Fresh fruit in season (apple, plum, etc)	70	
Coffee or tea	10	80 Cal
LUNCH		
Microwaveable Soup #18 (See Appendix B)	130	
String cheese (1 piece, any brand)	80	
Small whole-grain roll	80	
Coffee or tea	10	300 Cal
SNACK		
Handful unsalted mixed nuts	100	
Coffee or tea	10	110 Cal
DINNER		
Frozen Entree (See Appendix D)	340	
"Big-Bowl Salad"	150	
Fresh fruit in season (peach, plum, etc)	70	
Water with lemon wedge	15	565 Cal
SNACK		
Pop Popcorn Mini Bag	110	
Coffee or tea	10	120 Cal
		1510 Cal

Table from NoPaperPress eBook: *90-Day No-Cooking Diet - 1500 Calorie* with permission.

Table 11: Sample Weight Maintenance Daily Meal Plan

BREAKFAST	Calories	Totals
Grapefruit (½)	75	
Fried eggs (2 eggs) w Turkey bacon (2 slices)	270	
Whole wheat toast (2 slices +pat of butter)	250	
Coffee	10	605 Cal
MORNING SNACK		
Yogurt (6 oz nonfat, any flavor)	100	100 Cal
LUNCH		
Ham (3 oz) with mustard on 2 slices whole-grain bread	370	
Lettuce & tomato slices	20	
Vegetable soup (1 cup)	100	
Fresh fruit in season (apple, peach, plum, etc)	70	
Hot or iced tea	10	570 Cal
AFTERNOON SNACK		
Large handful of mixed nuts	150	
Coffee or tea	10	160 Cal
DINNER		
Chicken with Peppers & Onions (See Recipe)	250	
Sautéed red peppers with onions	70	
Green beans - steamed & mashed cauliflower	55	
Large tossed green salad with 2 Tbsp dressing	200	
Whole-grain bread (1 slice)	65	
Glass of wine (6 ounces)	150	
Water with lemon wedge	15	805 Cal
EVENING SNACK		
Three Ginger Snap cookies	240	
Coffee or tea	10	250 Cal
		2500

Table from NoPaperPress eBook: *Weight Maintenance - U.S. Edition* with permission.

Chicken with Peppers & Onions

4 boneless & skinless chicken breasts (about 5 oz each)

Coat the chicken breasts in a bottled barbeque sauce. Prepare medium-hot fire on well-oiled gas or charcoal grill. Place breasts on grill, turning them every 4 minutes, for 10 to 12 minutes, or until done. (To check if breasts are done, the meat should be moist and white with no sign of pink when you cut into breast.) Serve hot.

2 medium red peppers
1 medium onion

Place peppers and onions in pan with 2 Tbsp fat-free chicken stock. Sauté until stock is reduced. Spray pan lightly with non-stick cooking oil and sauté another 2 minutes. Salt and pepper to taste.

<u>Serves 4</u>. About 250 Calories per serving (for chicken only).

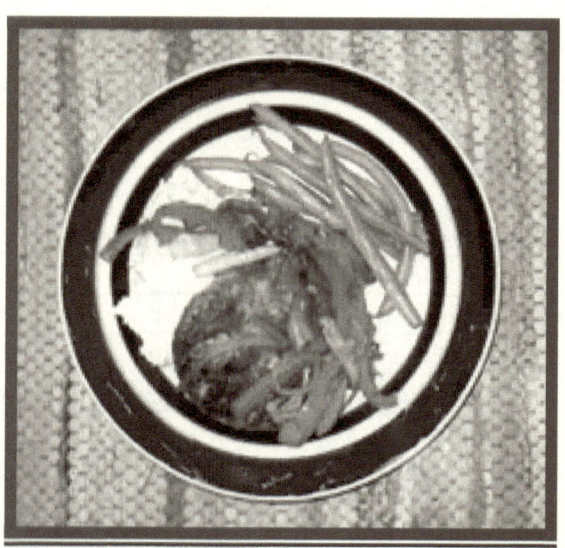

<u>Tip of the Day:</u> **Plan to be on a diet the rest of your life**. Not necessarily a weight reducing diet. At some point you'll want to just maintain your weight. But you will still need to continue to make good healthy food choices – and not slip back to your old eating habits.

Recipe from NoPaperPress eBook: *Weight Maintenance - U.S. Edition* with permission.

Appendix A Weight Loss Prediction Tables - Men

This appendix contains 36 Weight Loss Prediction Tables for Men. The tables cover men from 18 to 75 years, with heights ranging from 5' 0" to 6' 6", and activity levels from 0 to 4. Refer to the index shown in Table AA below to find the table that's right for you. Before choosing your personal Weight Loss Prediction table, you must determine your Activity Level see **Table 1** on page 17.

Age	Height	Activity Levels	Tables on Pages
18 - 35	5' 0" to 5' 5"	1 to 4	53 to 56
18 - 35	5' 6" to 5' 11"	1 to 4	57 to 60
18 - 35	6' 0" to 6' 6"	1 to 4	61 to 64
36 - 55	5' 0" to 5' 5"	0 to 3	65 to 68
36 - 55	5' 6" to 5' 11"	0 to 3	69 to 72
36 - 55	6' 0" to 6' 6"	0 to 3	73 to 76
56 - 75	5' 0" to 5' 5"	0 to 3	77 to 80
56 - 75	5' 6" to 5' 11"	0 to 3	81 to 84
56 - 75	6' 0" to 6' 6"	0 to 3	85 to 88

Table AA: 36 Weight Loss Prediction Tables for Men

Once you have selected the Weight Loss Prediction table that's appropriate for you, return to **Example 1** on page 35 for instruction on how to use the data in the table.

WEIGHT LOSS PREDICTION – MEN 18 to 35

Height: 5' 0" to 5' 5"   Activity Level 1

Weight Loss (lbs)	Diet Calories	Present Weight (lbs)							
		120	140	160	180	200	220	240	260
5	1200	20	17	14	12	11	10	9	8
	1500	30	23	18	15	13	12	11	10
	1800	58	36	26	21	17	15	13	11
	2100		83	45	31	24	19	16	14
10	1200	43	35	29	26	23	20	19	17
	1500	64	48	38	32	28	24	22	20
	1800	129	76	55	43	36	30	27	24
	2100		188	96	65	49	40	34	29
20	1200		73	61	53	47	42	39	36
	1500		103	81	67	58	51	46	41
	1800		172	119	92	75	64	56	49
	2100			222	143	106	85	71	61
30	1200		116	97	83	73	66	60	55
	1500		167	129	106	90	79	71	64
	1800		301	195	147	118	100	87	77
	2100			239	171	135	112	96	
40	1200			135	115	101	90	82	75
	1500			184	149	126	109	97	87
	1800			291	211	167	139	120	106
	2100				366	249	192	157	133
50	1200			178	150	131	116	105	96
	1500			249	197	164	142	125	112
	1800			287	222	183	156	136	
	2100				345	257	207	174	
60	1200	Values in table are		189	163	144	129	118	
	1500	time in days to		252	207	177	156	139	
	1800	lose weight		383	286	231	195	170	
	2100	indicated.			335	263	218		
70	1200				232	198	174	155	141
	1500				316	255	216	188	167
	1800					363	286	239	206
	2100						329	268	

Table A.1 Weight Loss Prediction: Men 18 to 35 5' 0" to 5' 5", Activity Level 1

WEIGHT LOSS PREDICTION – MEN   18 to 35

Height: 5' 0" to 5' 5"   Activity Level 2

Weight Loss (lbs)	Diet Calories	Present Weight (lbs)							
		120	140	160	180	200	220	240	260
5	1200	17	14	12	10	9	8	8	7
	1500	23	18	15	12	11	10	9	8
	1800	37	25	19	16	13	11	10	9
	2100	89	42	28	21	17	14	12	11
10	1200	35	29	25	21	19	17	16	14
	1500	49	38	31	26	23	20	18	16
	1800	80	53	40	33	28	24	21	19
	2100	215	92	59	44	35	29	25	22
20	1200		61	52	45	40	36	33	30
	1500		80	65	54	47	42	37	34
	1800		118	87	69	58	50	44	39
	2100		220	132	95	75	62	53	47
30	1200		97	81	70	62	55	50	46
	1500		130	103	86	74	65	58	52
	1800		198	141	110	91	78	68	61
	2100			224	155	119	98	83	72
40	1200			113	97	85	76	69	63
	1500			146	120	102	89	80	72
	1800			205	157	128	108	94	84
	2100			352	227	170	137	116	100
50	1200			149	126	110	98	88	81
	1500			195	158	133	116	103	92
	1800			285	210	168	141	122	108
	2100				319	230	182	151	130
60	1200	Values in table are time in days to lose weight indicated.			159	137	121	109	99
	1500				201	167	144	127	114
	1800				275	215	178	153	134
	2100					303	233	191	163
70	1200				194	167	146	131	119
	1500				250	205	175	154	137
	1800				355	269	219	186	162
	2100						293	236	198

Table A.2 Weight Loss Prediction: Men 18 to 35 5' 0" to 5' 5", Activity Level 2

WEIGHT LOSS PREDICTION – MEN   18 to 35

Height: 5' 0" to 5' 5"   Activity Level 3

Weight Loss (lbs)	Diet Calories	Present Weight (lbs)							
		120	140	160	180	200	220	240	260
5	1200	13	11	9	8	7	7	6	5
	1500	17	13	11	10	8	7	7	6
	1800	23	17	14	11	10	8	8	7
	2100	38	24	18	14	12	10	9	8
10	1200	28	23	20	17	15	14	13	11
	1500	36	28	23	20	17	15	14	13
	1800	50	36	29	24	20	18	16	14
	2100	82	51	37	29	24	21	18	16
20	1200		49	41	36	32	29	26	24
	1500		60	49	42	36	32	29	27
	1800		79	61	50	43	37	33	30
	2100		114	80	62	51	43	38	34
30	1200		77	65	56	49	44	40	37
	1500		96	78	65	57	50	45	41
	1800		129	98	79	67	58	51	46
	2100		196	131	100	81	68	59	52
40	1200			90	77	68	61	55	51
	1500			110	91	79	69	62	56
	1800			140	111	93	80	71	63
	2100			194	143	114	95	82	72
50	1200			119	101	88	79	71	65
	1500			146	120	102	90	80	72
	1800			190	148	122	104	91	81
	2100			277	194	151	125	107	93
60	1200	Values in table are time in days to lose weight indicated.			127	110	97	88	80
	1500				152	128	112	99	89
	1800				191	155	131	114	101
	2100				257	195	158	134	116
70	1200				155	133	117	105	95
	1500				188	157	135	119	107
	1800				241	191	160	138	121
	2100				340	246	195	163	141

Table A.3 Weight Loss Prediction: Men 18 to 35 5' 0" to 5' 5", Activity Level 3

WEIGHT LOSS PREDICTION – MEN 18 to 35

Height: 5' 0" to 5' 5"   Activity Level 4

Weight Loss (lbs)	Diet Calories	Present Weight (lbs)							
		120	140	160	180	200	220	240	260
5	1200	9	8	7	6	5	5	4	4
	1500	11	9	8	6	6	5	5	4
	1800	14	11	9	7	6	6	5	4
	2100	18	13	10	8	7	6	5	5
10	1200	20	16	14	12	11	10	9	8
	1500	23	19	16	14	12	11	10	9
	1800	29	22	18	15	13	12	11	10
	2100	38	27	21	18	15	13	12	10
20	1200		35	30	26	23	21	19	17
	1500		40	34	29	25	23	20	19
	1800		48	39	33	28	25	22	20
	2100		59	46	37	32	28	24	22
30	1200		55	46	40	36	32	29	27
	1500		64	53	45	39	35	32	29
	1800		77	62	51	44	39	35	31
	2100		97	73	59	50	43	38	34
40	1200			65	56	49	44	40	37
	1500			74	63	55	48	43	39
	1800			87	72	61	53	48	43
	2100			106	84	70	60	52	47
50	1200			85	73	64	57	51	47
	1500			98	82	71	63	56	51
	1800			117	95	80	69	61	55
	2100			144	111	92	78	68	60
60	1200	Values in table are		91	79	71	63	58	
	1500	time in days to		104	89	78	69	63	
	1800	lose weight		120	100	87	76	68	
	2100	indicated.		143	116	98	85	75	
70	1200			111	96	85	76	69	
	1500			128	108	94	83	75	
	1800			150	123	105	92	82	
	2100			182	144	120	103	90	

Table A.4 Weight Loss Prediction: Men 18 to 35 5' 0" to 5' 5", Activity Level 4

WEIGHT LOSS PREDICTION – MEN 18 to 35
Height: 5' 6" to 5' 11"   Activity Level 1

Weight Loss (lbs)	Diet Calories	Present Weight (lbs)							
		140	160	180	200	220	240	260	280
10	1200	31	27	23	21	19	17	16	15
	1500	42	34	29	25	22	20	18	17
	1800	62	46	37	32	27	24	22	20
	2100	120	73	53	42	35	30	26	23
20	1200		56	49	44	39	36	33	31
	1500		72	61	53	47	42	38	35
	1800		100	79	66	57	50	45	41
	2100		164	115	89	74	63	55	49
30	1200		88	76	67	61	55	51	47
	1500		114	95	82	72	65	59	54
	1800		162	126	104	89	78	70	63
	2100		285	189	143	116	98	85	75
40	1200			105	93	83	76	70	65
	1500			133	114	100	89	81	74
	1800			180	146	124	108	96	86
	2100			280	205	164	137	118	104
50	1200			137	120	107	97	89	82
	1500			175	148	129	115	104	95
	1800			242	193	162	140	124	111
	2100				279	217	179	153	134
60	1200				149	133	120	110	101
	1500				186	161	142	128	116
	1800				247	204	175	153	137
	2100				370	279	227	192	167
70	1200	Values in table are		181	160	144	131	120
	1500	time in days to		228	195	171	153	139
	1800	lose weight		309	251	213	185	165
	2100	indicated.			353	280	234	202
80	1200					189	169	154	141
	1500					233	203	181	163
	1800					304	254	220	195
	2100						342	282	241

Table A.5 Weight Loss Prediction: Men 18 - 35 5' 6" to 5' 11" Activity Level 1

WEIGHT LOSS PREDICTION – MEN 18 to 35

Height: 5' 6" to 5' 11"   Activity Level 2

Weight Loss (lbs)	Diet Calories	Present Weight (lbs)							
		140	160	180	200	220	240	260	280
10	1200	27	23	20	18	16	15	14	13
	1500	34	28	24	21	19	17	15	14
	1800	46	36	29	25	22	19	18	16
	2100	72	50	38	31	27	23	20	18
20	1200		48	42	37	34	31	28	26
	1500		59	50	44	39	35	32	29
	1800		76	62	53	46	41	36	33
	2100		109	82	66	56	48	43	38
30	1200		75	65	58	52	47	43	40
	1500		93	78	68	60	54	49	45
	1800		123	98	82	71	63	56	51
	2100		181	132	105	87	75	66	59
40	1200			90	79	71	65	59	55
	1500			109	94	83	74	67	62
	1800			139	115	99	87	77	70
	2100			191	149	122	104	91	81
50	1200			117	103	92	83	76	70
	1500			143	122	107	95	86	79
	1800			185	151	129	112	100	90
	2100			264	199	161	136	118	105
60	1200				127	113	102	93	86
	1500				153	133	118	106	97
	1800				192	161	140	124	111
	2100				258	205	171	147	130
70	1200	Values in table are time in days to lose weight indicated.			154	137	123	112	103
	1500				187	161	142	128	116
	1800				238	197	170	149	133
	2100				330	255	210	179	157
80	1200					162	144	131	120
	1500					192	168	150	136
	1800					238	202	177	157
	2100					314	254	214	186

Table A.6 Weight Loss Prediction: Men 18 - 35 5' 6" to 5' 11" Activity Level 2

WEIGHT LOSS PREDICTION – MEN 18 to 35

Height: 5' 6" to 5' 11" Activity Level 3

Weight Loss (lbs)	Diet Calories	Present Weight (lbs)							
		140	160	180	200	220	240	260	280
10	1200	21	18	16	14	13	12	11	10
	1500	26	22	19	16	15	13	12	11
	1800	33	26	22	19	17	15	13	12
	2100	44	33	27	22	19	17	15	14
20	1200		39	34	30	27	25	23	21
	1500		46	39	34	30	28	25	23
	1800		56	46	40	35	31	28	26
	2100		71	56	47	40	35	32	28
30	1200		60	53	47	42	38	35	33
	1500		72	61	53	47	43	39	36
	1800		89	73	62	54	48	43	39
	2100		115	90	74	63	55	49	44
40	1200			73	64	58	53	48	45
	1500			85	74	65	59	53	49
	1800			102	86	75	66	59	54
	2100			128	104	88	76	67	60
50	1200			95	83	74	67	62	57
	1500			111	96	84	75	68	63
	1800			135	113	97	86	77	69
	2100			172	137	115	99	87	78
60	1200				103	92	83	76	70
	1500				120	105	93	84	77
	1800				142	121	106	95	86
	2100				175	145	123	108	96
70	1200	Values in table are time in days to lose weight indicated.			125	111	100	91	83
	1500				146	127	112	101	92
	1800				175	148	129	114	103
	2100				220	178	150	131	116
80	1200					131	117	106	98
	1500					151	133	119	108
	1800					177	153	135	121
	2100					216	180	155	137

Table A.7 Weight Loss Prediction: Men 18 - 35 5' 6" to 5' 11" Activity Level 3

WEIGHT LOSS PREDICTION – MEN   18 to 35

Height: 5' 6" to 5' 11"   Activity Level 4

Weight Loss (lbs)	Diet Calories	Present Weight (lbs)							
		140	160	180	200	220	240	260	280
10	1200	16	13	12	10	9	9	8	7
	1500	18	15	13	11	10	9	9	8
	1800	21	17	15	13	11	10	9	8
	2100	25	20	17	14	12	11	10	9
20	1200		28	25	22	20	18	17	15
	1500		32	27	24	22	20	18	17
	1800		36	31	27	24	21	19	18
	2100		43	35	30	26	23	21	19
30	1200		44	39	34	31	28	26	24
	1500		50	43	38	34	30	28	26
	1800		58	49	42	37	33	30	27
	2100		68	56	47	41	36	33	30
40	1200			54	47	42	39	35	33
	1500			60	52	46	42	38	35
	1800			68	58	51	46	41	38
	2100			78	66	57	50	45	41
50	1200			70	61	55	50	45	42
	1500			78	68	60	54	49	45
	1800			89	76	66	59	53	48
	2100			104	86	74	65	58	52
60	1200				76	68	61	56	51
	1500				85	74	66	60	55
	1800				95	82	73	65	59
	2100				109	92	81	71	64
70	1200	Values in table are time in days to lose weight indicated.			92	82	73	67	61
	1500				103	90	80	72	66
	1800				117	100	88	79	71
	2100				134	113	98	86	77
80	1200					96	86	78	72
	1500					107	94	85	77
	1800					119	104	93	84
	2100					136	116	102	91

Table A.8 Weight Loss Prediction: Men 18 - 35 5' 6" to 5' 11" Activity Level 4

WEIGHT LOSS PREDICTION – MEN 18 to 35

Height: 6' 0" to 6' 6"   Activity Level 1

Weight Loss (lbs)	Diet Calories	Present Weight (lbs)							
		160	180	200	220	240	260	280	300
10	1200	25	22	20	18	16	15	14	13
	1500	31	27	23	21	19	17	16	15
	1800	41	34	29	25	22	20	18	17
	2100	61	46	37	31	27	24	22	20
20	1200		46	41	37	34	31	29	27
	1500		56	49	43	39	36	33	31
	1800		71	60	52	46	42	38	35
	2100		99	79	66	57	50	45	41
30	1200		71	63	57	52	48	45	42
	1500		87	76	67	61	55	51	47
	1800		113	95	82	72	65	59	54
	2100		161	126	104	89	78	69	63
40	1200			87	78	72	66	61	57
	1500			105	93	83	76	70	64
	1800			132	113	99	89	80	74
	2100			179	146	123	108	96	86
50	1200			112	101	92	84	78	73
	1500			137	120	107	97	89	82
	1800			174	148	129	114	103	94
	2100			240	192	161	139	123	111
60	1200				125	113	103	96	89
	1500				149	132	120	109	101
	1800				185	160	142	127	116
	2100				245	203	174	153	137
70	1200	Values in table are			150	135	124	114	106
	1500	time in days to			180	160	144	131	120
	1800	lose weight			227	195	171	153	139
	2100	indicated.			307	250	212	185	164
80	1200					159	145	133	124
	1500					189	169	153	141
	1800					232	203	180	163
	2100					303	254	219	194

Table A.9 Weight Loss Prediction: Men, 18 - 35, 6' 0" to 6' 6" Activity Level 1

WEIGHT LOSS PREDICTION – MEN 18 to 35

Height: 6' 0" to 6' 6"   Activity Level 2

Weight Loss (lbs)	Diet Calories	Present Weight (lbs)							
		160	180	200	220	240	260	280	300
10	1200	21	19	17	15	14	13	12	11
	1500	26	22	20	18	16	15	13	12
	1800	32	27	23	20	18	17	15	14
	2100	44	34	29	24	21	19	17	16
20	1200		39	35	32	29	27	25	23
	1500		47	41	36	33	30	28	26
	1800		57	49	43	38	34	31	29
	2100		74	60	51	45	40	36	33
30	1200		61	54	49	45	41	39	36
	1500		73	64	57	51	47	43	40
	1800		90	76	66	59	53	48	44
	2100		118	95	80	70	62	55	50
40	1200			75	68	62	57	53	49
	1500			88	78	70	64	59	54
	1800			106	92	81	73	66	61
	2100			134	112	96	85	76	69
50	1200			97	87	79	72	67	62
	1500			114	101	90	82	75	69
	1800			139	119	105	94	85	78
	2100			179	147	126	110	98	89
60	1200				107	97	89	82	76
	1500				125	111	101	92	85
	1800				149	130	116	105	96
	2100				186	157	137	121	109
70	1200	Values in table are			129	117	106	98	91
	1500	time in days to			151	134	121	110	101
	1800	lose weight			182	158	140	126	114
	2100	indicated.			230	192	166	146	131
80	1200					137	125	115	106
	1500					158	142	129	118
	1800					188	165	148	134
	2100					231	197	173	154

Table A.10 Weight Loss Prediction: Men 18 - 35 6' 0" to 6' 6" Activity Level 2

WEIGHT LOSS PREDICTION – MEN 18 to 35
Height: 6' 0" to 6' 6"   Activity Level 3

Weight Loss (lbs)	Diet Calories	Present Weight (lbs)							
		160	180	200	220	240	260	280	300
10	1200	17	15	14	12	11	11	10	9
	1500	20	18	16	14	13	12	11	10
	1800	24	21	18	16	14	13	12	11
	2100	30	25	21	18	16	14	13	12
20	1200		32	29	26	24	22	20	19
	1500		37	33	29	26	24	22	21
	1800		43	37	33	29	27	24	23
	2100		52	44	38	33	30	27	25
30	1200		50	45	40	37	34	31	29
	1500		58	51	45	41	37	34	32
	1800		68	58	51	46	41	38	35
	2100		83	69	59	52	46	42	38
40	1200			62	55	50	46	43	40
	1500			70	62	56	51	47	43
	1800			81	71	63	57	52	48
	2100			97	82	72	64	58	52
50	1200			79	71	65	59	55	51
	1500			91	80	72	65	60	56
	1800			106	92	81	73	66	61
	2100			127	107	93	82	74	67
60	1200				88	80	73	67	62
	1500				100	89	81	74	68
	1800				115	101	90	82	75
	2100				135	116	102	91	83
70	1200	Values in table are			106	96	87	80	74
	1500	time in days to			120	107	97	88	81
	1800	lose weight			139	122	108	98	89
	2100	indicated.			166	141	123	110	99
80	1200					112	102	94	87
	1500					126	114	103	95
	1800					145	128	115	105
	2100					169	147	130	117

Table A.11 Weight Loss Prediction: Men, 18 - 35, 6' 0" to 6' 6", Activity Level 3

WEIGHT LOSS PREDICTION – MEN 18 to 35

Height: 6' 0" to 6' 6"   Activity Level 4

Weight Loss (lbs)	Diet Calories	Present Weight (lbs)							
		160	180	200	220	240	260	280	300
10	1200	13	11	10	9	8	8	7	7
	1500	14	13	11	10	9	8	8	7
	1800	16	14	12	11	10	9	8	8
	2100	19	16	14	12	11	10	9	8
20	1200		24	21	19	18	16	15	14
	1500		26	23	21	19	17	16	15
	1800		30	26	23	21	19	17	16
	2100		34	29	25	22	20	18	17
30	1200		37	33	30	27	25	23	22
	1500		41	36	33	29	27	25	23
	1800		46	40	36	32	29	27	25
	2100		53	45	39	35	31	29	26
40	1200			46	41	37	34	32	30
	1500			50	45	40	37	34	31
	1800			56	49	44	40	36	34
	2100			63	54	48	43	39	36
50	1200			59	53	48	44	41	38
	1500			65	58	52	47	43	40
	1800			73	64	57	51	47	43
	2100			82	71	62	56	50	46
60	1200				66	59	54	50	46
	1500				72	64	58	53	49
	1800				79	70	63	57	53
	2100				88	77	69	62	57
70	1200	Values in table are			79	71	65	60	55
	1500	time in days to			87	77	70	64	59
	1800	lose weight			96	85	76	69	63
	2100	indicated.			108	94	83	75	68
80	1200					84	76	70	64
	1500					91	82	75	69
	1800					100	89	81	74
	2100					111	98	88	80

Table A.12 Weight Loss Prediction: Men 18 - 35 6' 0" to 6' 6" Activity Level 4

WEIGHT LOSS PREDICTION – MEN 36 to 55

Height: 5' 0" to 5' 5"   Activity Level 0

Weight Loss (lbs)	Diet Calories	Present Weight (lbs)							
		120	140	160	180	200	220	240	260
5	1200	25	20	17	15	13	12	11	10
	1500	42	30	23	19	16	14	13	12
	1800	123	56	37	28	22	19	16	14
	2100			89	50	35	27	22	19
10	1200	52	42	35	30	27	24	22	20
	1500	89	62	48	40	34	30	26	24
	1800	300	122	78	58	46	39	33	29
	2100			200	106	73	56	46	39
20	1200		89	74	63	56	50	45	41
	1500		136	103	84	71	62	55	49
	1800		294	173	125	98	82	70	61
	2100				245	160	120	96	81
30	1200		142	116	99	86	77	70	64
	1500		226	166	133	111	96	85	76
	1800			296	203	157	128	109	95
	2100					266	193	153	127
40	1200			163	137	119	106	95	87
	1500			240	188	155	133	117	105
	1800				299	224	180	152	132
	2100						280	216	177
50	1200			216	179	155	136	123	111
	1500			330	250	204	174	152	135
	1800					302	239	199	171
	2100						386	290	234
60	1200	Values in table are time in days to lose weight indicated.			226	193	169	151	137
	1500				324	259	218	189	167
	1800					398	306	251	214
	2100							377	298
70	1200				279	236	205	182	164
	1500					322	267	229	201
	1800						384	309	261
	2100								371

Table A.13 Weight Loss Prediction: Men 36 to 55, 5' 0" to 5' 5", Activity Level 0

WEIGHT LOSS PREDICTION – MEN   36 to 55

Height: 5' 0" to 5' 5"   Activity Level 1

Weight Loss (lbs)	Diet Calories	Present Weight (lbs)							
		120	140	160	180	200	220	240	260
5	1200	23	18	15	13	12	11	10	9
	1500	35	26	20	17	15	13	11	10
	1800	80	44	30	23	19	16	14	12
	2100		139	58	37	28	22	18	16
10	1200	47	38	32	27	24	22	20	18
	1500	75	54	42	35	30	26	24	21
	1800	182	93	64	49	40	34	29	26
	2100		356	127	79	58	46	38	33
20	1200		80	67	57	51	45	41	38
	1500		117	90	74	63	55	49	44
	1800		217	140	104	84	70	61	54
	2100			313	177	125	97	80	68
30	1200		128	105	90	79	70	63	58
	1500		193	145	117	99	86	76	68
	1800			234	169	133	111	95	83
	2100				304	204	155	126	106
40	1200			147	125	108	96	87	79
	1500			208	165	138	119	105	94
	1800			357	245	189	155	132	115
	2100					302	222	177	148
50	1200			195	163	141	124	112	102
	1500			283	219	181	154	135	121
	1800				339	253	204	172	149
	2100						302	236	195
60	1200	Values in table are		205	176	154	138	125
	1500	time in days to		282	229	193	168	150
	1800	lose weight			329	260	216	186
	2100	indicated.					303	246
70	1200				253	214	187	166	150
	1500				358	283	236	204	180
	1800						324	265	226
	2100							382	304

Table A.14 Weight Loss Prediction: Men 36 to 55, 5' 0" to 5' 5", Activity Level 1

WEIGHT LOSS PREDICTION – MEN 36 to 55

Height: 5' 0" to 5' 5"   Activity Level 2

Weight Loss (lbs)	Diet Calories	Present Weight (lbs)							
		120	140	160	180	200	220	240	260
5	1200	18	15	13	11	10	9	8	7
	1500	26	20	16	13	12	10	9	8
	1800	45	29	22	17	14	12	11	10
	2100	153	54	33	24	19	16	13	12
10	1200	38	31	26	23	20	18	17	15
	1500	55	41	33	28	24	21	19	17
	1800	98	61	45	36	30	26	23	20
	2100		118	70	50	39	32	28	24
20	1200		66	55	48	42	38	34	31
	1500		89	71	59	51	44	40	26
	1800		137	98	76	63	54	47	42
	2100		303	158	109	84	68	58	50
30	1200		105	87	75	65	58	53	48
	1500		145	112	93	79	69	62	56
	1800		235	159	122	99	84	73	65
	2100			277	180	134	108	91	78
40	1200			122	103	90	80	73	66
	1500			160	130	110	95	85	76
	1800			235	174	140	117	101	90
	2100				268	193	153	127	109
50	1200			161	135	117	104	93	85
	1500			216	172	144	124	109	98
	1800			333	236	186	154	132	116
	2100				387	264	203	166	141
60	1200	Values in table are	time in days to lose weight		170	146	129	115	105
	1500				219	181	155	136	121
	1800				312	238	194	165	144
	2100	indicated.				352	262	211	177
70	1200				209	178	155	139	125
	1500				275	223	188	164	146
	1800					300	240	201	174
	2100						333	262	217

Table A.15 Weight Loss Prediction: Men 36 to 55, 5' 0" to 5' 5", Activity Level 2

WEIGHT LOSS PREDICTION – MEN 36 to 55

Height: 5' 0" to 5' 5"   Activity Level 3

Weight Loss (lbs)	Diet Calories	Present Weight (lbs)							
		120	140	160	180	200	220	240	260
5	1200	14	12	10	9	8	7	6	6
	1500	19	14	12	10	9	8	7	6
	1800	26	19	15	12	10	9	8	7
	2100	46	27	19	15	12	11	9	8
10	1200	30	24	21	18	16	14	13	12
	1500	39	30	25	21	18	16	15	13
	1800	56	40	31	25	22	19	17	15
	2100	101	58	41	32	26	22	19	17
20	1200		52	43	38	33	30	27	25
	1500		65	52	44	38	34	31	28
	1800		87	66	54	45	39	35	31
	2100		132	89	68	55	46	40	36
30	1200		82	68	59	52	46	42	38
	1500		104	83	70	60	53	47	43
	1800		144	106	85	71	61	54	48
	2100		234	148	109	87	73	63	55
40	1200			96	82	72	64	58	53
	1500			118	97	83	73	65	59
	1800			153	120	99	85	74	66
	2100			222	158	124	102	87	76
50	1200			126	106	93	82	74	67
	1500			157	128	108	94	84	75
	1800			210	161	131	111	97	86
	2100			323	216	165	134	114	99
60	1200	Values in table are			134	115	102	91	83
	1500	time in days to			162	136	118	104	93
	1800	lose weight			208	166	139	120	106
	2100	indicated.			390	213	171	143	123
70	1200				164	140	123	110	100
	1500				202	167	143	125	112
	1800				264	206	171	146	128
	2100				392	272	212	175	150

Table A.16 Weight Loss Prediction: Men 36 to 55, 5' 0" to 5' 5", Activity Level 3

WEIGHT LOSS PREDICTION – MEN 36 to 55
Height: 5' 6" to 5' 11"   Activity Level 0

Weight Loss (lbs)	Diet Calories	Present Weight (lbs)							
		140	160	180	200	220	240	260	280
10	1200	39	33	28	25	23	21	19	18
	1500	56	44	37	32	28	25	23	21
	1800	99	68	52	42	36	31	27	25
	2100		143	87	63	50	41	35	31
20	1200		69	59	52	47	43	39	36
	1500		94	77	66	58	52	47	43
	1800		148	111	89	75	65	57	51
	2100		360	195	136	105	86	74	64
30	1200		108	92	81	73	66	61	56
	1500		150	122	103	90	80	72	66
	1800		248	179	141	117	101	89	79
	2100			339	224	169	137	115	100
40	1200			128	112	100	90	83	76
	1500			172	144	124	110	99	90
	1800			259	200	164	140	122	109
	2100				332	242	192	161	138
50	1200			168	145	129	116	106	98
	1500			228	188	161	142	127	115
	1800			359	268	216	182	158	140
	2100					330	256	211	180
60	1200				181	160	143	130	120
	1500				238	202	176	157	142
	1800				349	275	229	197	174
	2100						329	267	225
70	1200	Values in table are time in days to lose weight indicated.			221	193	172	156	143
	1500				294	247	213	189	170
	1800					343	281	240	210
	2100							330	275
80	1200					229	203	183	167
	1500					296	254	223	200
	1800						340	287	249
	2100								331

Table A.17 Weight Loss Prediction: Men 36 - 55 5' 6" - 5' 11" Activity Level 0

WEIGHT LOSS PREDICTION – MEN 36 to 55

Height: 5' 6" to 5' 11"   Activity Level 1

Weight Loss (lbs)	Diet Calories	Present Weight (lbs)							
		140	160	180	200	220	240	260	280
10	1200	35	30	26	23	21	19	17	16
	1500	49	39	33	28	25	22	20	19
	1800	80	57	44	36	31	27	24	22
	2100	212	102	68	51	41	35	30	27
20	1200		63	54	48	43	39	36	33
	1500		83	69	59	52	46	42	38
	1800		123	94	77	65	57	50	45
	2100		239	149	110	88	73	63	55
30	1200		98	85	74	67	60	55	51
	1500		132	108	92	81	72	65	59
	1800		203	151	122	102	88	78	70
	2100			252	178	139	115	98	86
40	1200			117	103	92	83	76	70
	1500			152	128	111	99	89	81
	1800			218	172	143	122	108	96
	2100			389	260	198	161	136	119
50	1200			153	133	118	106	97	89
	1500			202	168	145	128	114	104
	1800			298	229	187	159	139	124
	2100				362	266	213	178	154
60	1200				166	146	131	119	110
	1500				212	181	158	141	128
	1800				295	237	200	173	154
	2100					348	272	224	192
70	1200	Values in table are time in days to lose weight indicated.			202	177	158	143	131
	1500				261	220	192	170	153
	1800				375	294	245	210	185
	2100					340	276	234
80	1200					209	186	168	153
	1500					264	228	201	180
	1800					361	295	251	219
	2100						335	280

Table A.18 Weight Loss Prediction: Men 36 - 55, 5' 6" to 5' 11"Activity Level 1

WEIGHT LOSS PREDICTION – MEN 36 to 55

Height: 5' 6" to 5' 11"   Activity Level 2

Weight Loss (lbs)	Diet Calories	Present Weight (lbs)							
		140	160	180	200	220	240	260	280
10	1200	29	25	22	19	17	16	15	14
	1500	38	31	26	23	20	18	17	15
	1800	55	41	33	28	24	21	19	17
	2100	97	61	45	36	30	26	23	20
20	1200		52	45	40	36	33	30	28
	1500		66	55	48	42	38	34	32
	1800		89	71	59	51	45	40	36
	2100		137	98	77	63	54	47	42
30	1200		82	71	63	56	51	47	43
	1500		105	87	75	66	59	53	49
	1800		145	113	93	79	69	62	56
	2100		234	160	123	100	85	74	65
40	1200			98	86	77	70	64	59
	1500			122	104	91	81	73	67
	1800			160	130	110	96	85	77
	2100			236	175	141	118	102	90
50	1200			128	112	99	90	82	75
	1500			161	135	118	104	94	85
	1800			216	172	144	124	110	98
	2100			333	237	187	155	133	116
60	1200				139	123	110	100	92
	1500				170	147	129	116	105
	1800				220	182	155	136	122
	2100				313	239	195	166	145
70	1200	Values in table are time in days to lose weight indicated.			169	148	133	120	110
	1500				209	178	156	139	126
	1800				276	224	189	165	146
	2100					301	241	203	175
80	1200					176	156	141	129
	1500					213	185	164	148
	1800					271	227	196	173
	2100					377	294	243	209

Table A.19 Weight Loss Prediction: Men 36 - 55, 5' 6" to 5' 11" Activity Level 2

WEIGHT LOSS PREDICTION – MEN 36 to 55

Height: 5' 6" to 5' 11"   Activity Level 3

Weight Loss (lbs)	Diet Calories	Present Weight (lbs)							
		140	160	180	200	220	240	260	280
10	1200	23	20	17	15	14	13	12	11
	1500	29	24	20	18	16	14	13	12
	1800	37	29	24	21	18	16	14	13
	2100	52	38	30	25	21	18	16	15
20	1200		42	36	32	29	26	24	22
	1500		50	42	37	33	29	27	25
	1800		62	51	43	38	33	30	27
	2100		82	64	52	44	38	34	31
30	1200		65	57	50	45	41	37	34
	1500		79	66	57	51	46	41	38
	1800		100	80	68	59	52	46	42
	2100		135	102	82	69	60	53	47
40	1200			78	69	62	56	51	47
	1500			93	80	70	63	57	52
	1800			113	95	81	71	64	58
	2100			146	116	97	83	73	65
50	1200			102	89	79	72	65	60
	1500			122	104	91	81	73	66
	1800			151	124	106	92	82	74
	2100			199	154	127	108	95	84
60	1200				111	98	88	80	74
	1500				130	113	100	90	82
	1800				157	133	115	102	92
	2100				199	161	136	118	104
70	1200	Values in table are time in days to lose weight indicated.			135	119	106	96	88
	1500				159	137	121	108	98
	1800				195	162	140	123	110
	2100				252	199	166	143	126
80	1200					141	125	113	103
	1500					163	143	127	115
	1800					195	166	146	130
	2100					243	200	170	149

Table A.20 Weight Loss Prediction: Men 36 - 55 5' 6" to 5' 11" Activity Level 3

WEIGHT LOSS PREDICTION – MEN 36 to 55

Height: 6' 0" to 6' 6"   Activity Level 0

Weight Loss (lbs)	Diet Calories	Present Weight (lbs)							
		160	180	200	220	240	260	280	300
10	1200	29	25	23	21	19	17	16	15
	1500	38	32	28	25	22	20	19	17
	1800	54	43	36	31	27	24	22	20
	2100	93	64	50	41	35	30	27	24
20	1200		53	47	43	39	36	33	31
	1500		67	58	51	46	42	39	36
	1800		91	75	64	56	50	46	42
	2100		141	106	86	72	63	55	50
30	1200		82	73	66	60	55	51	48
	1500		105	90	80	71	65	59	55
	1800		145	118	100	88	78	70	64
	2100		234	171	136	113	98	86	77
40	1200			101	90	82	76	70	65
	1500			125	110	98	89	81	75
	1800			166	140	121	107	96	88
	2100			247	192	159	136	119	106
50	1200			130	116	105	97	89	83
	1500			164	142	126	114	104	96
	1800			220	183	157	138	124	112
	2100			340	257	209	177	154	136
60	1200				144	130	119	109	102
	1500				177	156	140	128	117
	1800				231	197	172	153	138
	2100				334	265	222	191	169
70	1200	Values in table are			173	156	142	131	121
	1500	time in days to			215	189	169	153	140
	1800	lose weight			285	240	208	184	166
	2100	indicated.				330	272	233	204
80	1200					183	166	153	141
	1500					224	199	179	164
	1800					288	247	218	195
	2100						328	278	242

Table A.21 Weight Loss Prediction: Men 36 to 55, 6' 0" to 6' 6", Activity Level 0

WEIGHT LOSS PREDICTION – MEN 36 to 55

Height: 6' 0" to 6' 6"   Activity Level 1

Weight Loss (lbs)	Diet Calories	Present Weight (lbs)							
		160	180	200	220	240	260	280	300
10	1200	27	23	21	19	17	16	15	14
	1500	34	29	25	22	20	18	17	16
	1800	46	37	32	27	24	22	20	18
	2100	73	53	42	35	30	26	23	21
20	1200		49	44	39	36	33	31	29
	1500		61	53	47	42	38	35	33
	1800		79	66	57	50	45	41	37
	2100		115	89	74	63	55	49	44
30	1200		76	67	61	55	51	47	45
	1500		95	82	72	65	59	54	50
	1800		126	104	89	78	70	63	58
	2100		189	143	116	98	85	75	68
40	1200			93	83	76	70	65	60
	1500			114	100	89	81	74	68
	1800			146	124	108	96	86	79
	2100			205	164	137	118	104	93
50	1200			120	107	97	89	82	77
	1500			148	129	115	104	95	87
	1800			193	162	140	124	111	101
	2100			279	217	179	153	134	120
60	1200				133	120	110	101	94
	1500				161	142	128	116	107
	1800				204	175	153	137	124
	2100				279	227	192	167	148
70	1200	Values in table are time in days to lose weight indicated.			160	144	131	120	112
	1500				195	171	153	139	128
	1800				251	213	185	165	149
	2100				353	280	234	202	179
80	1200					169	154	141	130
	1500					203	181	163	149
	1800					254	220	195	175
	2100					342	282	241	211

Table A.22 Weight Loss Prediction: Men 36 to 55, 6' 0" - 6' 6" Activity Level 1

WEIGHT LOSS PREDICTION – MEN   36 to 55
Height: 6' 0" to 6' 6"   Activity Level 2

Weight Loss (lbs)	Diet Calories	Present Weight (lbs)							
		160	180	200	220	240	260	280	300
10	1200	23	20	18	16	15	14	13	12
	1500	28	24	21	19	17	15	14	13
	1800	36	29	25	22	19	18	16	15
	2100	50	38	31	27	23	20	18	17
20	1200		42	37	34	31	28	26	24
	1500		50	44	39	35	32	29	27
	1800		62	53	46	41	36	33	30
	2100		82	66	56	48	43	38	35
30	1200		65	58	52	47	44	40	38
	1500		78	68	60	54	49	45	42
	1800		98	82	71	63	56	51	47
	2100		132	105	87	75	66	59	54
40	1200			79	71	65	59	55	51
	1500			94	83	74	67	62	57
	1800			115	99	87	77	70	64
	2100			149	122	104	91	81	73
50	1200			103	92	83	76	70	65
	1500			122	107	95	86	79	73
	1800			151	129	112	100	90	82
	2100			199	161	136	118	105	94
60	1200				113	102	93	86	80
	1500				133	118	106	97	89
	1800				161	140	124	111	101
	2100				205	171	147	130	116
70	1200	Values in table are		137	123	112	103	95
	1500	time in days to		161	142	128	116	107
	1800	lose weight		197	170	149	133	121
	2100	indicated.		255	210	179	157	140
80	1200					144	131	120	111
	1500					168	150	136	125
	1800					202	177	157	142
	2100					254	214	186	165

Table A.23 Weight Loss Prediction: Men, 36 - 55, 6' 0" - 6' 6" Activity Level 2

WEIGHT LOSS PREDICTION – MEN 36 to 55
Height: 6' 0" to 6' 6"   Activity Level 3

Weight Loss (lbs)	Diet Calories	Present Weight (lbs)							
		160	180	200	220	240	260	280	300
10	1200	18	16	14	13	12	11	10	9
	1500	22	19	16	15	13	12	11	10
	1800	26	22	19	17	15	13	12	11
	2100	33	27	22	19	17	15	14	12
20	1200		34	30	27	25	23	21	20
	1500		39	34	30	28	25	23	21
	1800		46	40	35	31	28	26	24
	2100		55	47	40	35	32	28	26
30	1200		53	47	42	38	35	33	30
	1500		61	53	47	43	39	36	33
	1800		73	62	54	48	43	39	36
	2100		90	74	63	55	49	44	40
40	1200			64	58	53	48	45	41
	1500			74	65	59	53	49	45
	1800			86	75	66	59	54	50
	2100			104	88	76	67	60	55
50	1200			83	74	67	62	57	53
	1500			96	84	75	68	63	58
	1800			113	97	86	77	69	64
	2100			137	115	99	87	78	71
60	1200				92	83	76	70	65
	1500				105	93	84	77	71
	1800				121	106	95	86	78
	2100				145	123	108	96	87
70	1200	Values in table are			111	100	91	83	77
	1500	time in days to			127	112	101	92	85
	1800	lose weight			148	129	114	103	93
	2100	indicated.			178	150	131	116	104
80	1200					117	106	98	90
	1500					133	119	108	99
	1800					153	135	121	110
	2100					180	155	137	123

Table A.24 Weight Loss Prediction: Men 36 to 55, 6' 0" to 6' 6", Activity Level 3

WEIGHT LOSS PREDICTION – MEN 56 to 75

Height: 5' 0" to 5' 5"   Activity Level 0

Weight Loss (lbs)	Diet Calories	Present Weight (lbs)							
		120	140	160	180	200	220	240	260
5	1200	29	23	19	16	14	13	11	10
	1500	53	36	27	22	18	16	14	13
	1800	329	81	47	34	26	22	18	16
	2100			181	71	45	33	26	22
10	1200	60	47	39	33	29	26	24	22
	1500	115	75	56	45	38	33	29	26
	1800		181	100	70	54	44	38	33
	2100				155	95	68	54	45
20	1200		101	82	70	61	54	49	45
	1500		166	121	96	80	69	60	54
	1800			229	153	116	94	79	69
	2100				388	212	148	115	94
30	1200		162	130	109	95	84	75	69
	1500		281	196	152	125	107	94	84
	1800			254	187	149	124	107
	2100				368	243	184	148
40	1200			183	152	131	115	103	94
	1500			287	217	176	149	130	115
	1800				383	269	210	174	148
	2100					361	263	209
50	1200			244	200	170	149	133	120
	1500			292	233	195	168	148
	1800				370	281	228	193
	2100					358	278
60	1200	Values in table are time in days to lose weight indicated.			253	213	185	165	149
	1500				383	297	245	210	184
	1800					364	290	243
	2100						358
70	1200				314	261	225	198	178
	1500					373	302	256	223
	1800						361	298
	2100						

Table A.25 Weight Loss Prediction: Men 56 to 75, 5' 0" to 5' 5", Activity Level 0

WEIGHT LOSS PREDICTION – MEN 56 to 75

Height: 5' 0" to 5' 5"   Activity Level 1

Weight Loss (lbs)	Diet Calories	Present Weight (lbs)							
		120	140	160	180	200	220	240	260
5	1200	26	20	17	14	13	11	10	9
	1500	43	30	23	19	16	14	12	11
	1800	134	57	37	27	22	18	16	14
	2100			88	48	34	26	21	18
10	1200	54	42	35	30	26	24	21	20
	1500	92	63	48	39	33	29	26	23
	1800	341	125	78	57	45	38	32	28
	2100			199	103	70	54	44	37
20	1200		90	74	63	55	49	44	40
	1500		138	103	83	70	61	54	48
	1800		306	174	123	96	79	68	59
	2100				240	155	115	92	77
30	1200		144	116	98	85	76	68	62
	1500		231	167	132	110	94	83	74
	1800			299	202	154	125	106	92
	2100					258	186	146	121
40	1200			164	137	118	104	94	85
	1500			242	187	154	131	115	102
	1800				298	220	176	148	127
	2100					395	270	208	170
50	1200			218	179	154	135	120	109
	1500			335	251	202	171	148	132
	1800				299	234	193	166	
	2100					374	279	224	
60	1200	Values in table are			227	192	168	149	134
	1500	time in days to			326	258	215	185	163
	1800	lose weight				395	300	245	207
	2100	indicated.						363	286
70	1200				281	235	203	179	161
	1500					321	264	225	197
	1800						378	302	253
	2100								356

Table A.26 Weight Loss Prediction: Men 56 to 75, 5' 0" to 5' 5", Activity Level 1

WEIGHT LOSS PREDICTION – MEN 56 to 75

Height: 5' 0" to 5' 5"   Activity Level 2

Weight Loss (lbs)	Diet Calories	Present Weight (lbs)							
		120	140	160	180	200	220	240	260
5	1200	20	16	14	12	10	9	8	8
	1500	30	22	18	15	13	11	10	9
	1800	58	35	25	19	16	14	12	10
	2100		76	41	28	21	17	15	13
10	1200	43	34	28	25	22	19	18	16
	1500	64	47	37	31	26	23	20	18
	1800	129	73	52	40	33	28	25	22
	2100		174	87	59	45	36	30	26
20	1200		72	60	51	45	40	36	33
	1500		101	78	64	55	48	43	38
	1800		167	113	86	70	59	51	45
	2100			204	130	96	77	64	55
30	1200		115	94	80	70	62	56	51
	1500		166	125	102	86	75	66	59
	1800		297	187	138	111	93	80	70
	2100			378	218	156	122	101	86
40	1200			133	112	97	86	77	70
	1500			180	143	120	103	91	81
	1800			281	200	157	129	111	97
	2100				334	227	174	141	120
50	1200			176	146	126	111	99	90
	1500			244	190	157	134	118	105
	1800				274	209	170	144	126
	2100					315	233	187	156
60	1200	Values in table are time in days to lose weight indicated.			185	157	138	123	111
	1500				245	199	168	146	130
	1800				368	270	216	181	156
	2100					304	238	197
70	1200				228	192	167	148	133
	1500				309	246	205	177	157
	1800					344	268	222	190
	2100						392	298	242

Table A.27 Weight Loss Prediction: Men 56 to 75, 5' 0" to 5' 5", Activity Level 2

WEIGHT LOSS PREDICTION – MEN 56 to 75

Height: 5' 0" to 5' 5"   Activity Level 3

Weight Loss (lbs)	Diet Calories	Present Weight (lbs)							
		120	140	160	180	200	220	240	260
5	1200	15	12	11	9	8	7	7	6
	1500	21	16	13	11	9	8	7	7
	1800	31	21	16	13	11	10	8	8
	2100	59	32	22	17	14	11	10	9
10	1200	32	26	22	19	17	15	14	13
	1500	43	33	27	23	19	17	15	14
	1800	66	45	34	27	23	20	18	16
	2100	136	69	46	35	28	24	21	18
20	1200		55	46	40	35	31	29	26
	1500		71	57	47	41	36	32	29
	1800		98	73	58	49	42	37	33
	2100		160	102	76	60	50	43	38
30	1200		88	73	62	55	49	44	40
	1500		115	90	75	64	56	50	45
	1800		164	118	93	77	66	57	51
	2100		296	171	123	96	79	68	59
40	1200			102	87	76	67	61	55
	1500			128	105	89	77	69	62
	1800			171	132	108	91	79	70
	2100			263	178	136	111	94	82
50	1200			135	113	98	87	78	71
	1500			172	138	116	100	89	80
	1800			238	177	142	119	103	91
	2100				247	183	147	123	106
60	1200	Values in table are time in days to lose weight indicated.			143	122	108	96	87
	1500				176	146	125	11	98
	1800				230	181	150	129	113
	2100				339	239	187	155	132
70	1200				175	149	130	116	104
	1500				220	179	152	133	118
	1800				296	226	184	157	136
	2100					308	234	191	161

Table A.28 Weight Loss Prediction: Men 56 to 75, 5' 0" to 5' 5", Activity Level 3

WEIGHT LOSS PREDICTION – MEN   56 to 75

Height: 5' 6" to 5' 11"   Activity Level 0

Weight Loss (lbs)	Diet Calories	Present Weight (lbs)							
		140	160	180	200	220	240	260	280
10	1200	44	36	31	28	25	22	21	19
	1500	66	51	42	35	31	27	25	22
	1800	137	85	62	49	41	35	31	27
	2100		250	119	79	60	48	40	35
20	1200		76	65	57	51	46	42	39
	1500		109	88	74	64	57	51	46
	1800		189	133	104	85	73	64	57
	2100			280	175	128	102	85	73
30	1200		120	102	89	79	71	65	60
	1500		175	139	116	100	88	79	71
	1800		327	218	166	135	114	99	88
	2100				294	208	162	133	114
40	1200			142	123	109	98	89	82
	1500			197	162	138	121	108	98
	1800			323	238	190	159	137	121
	2100					304	231	187	158
50	1200			186	160	141	126	114	105
	1500			264	213	180	157	139	126
	1800				323	252	208	178	156
	2100						310	247	207
60	1200				200	175	156	141	129
	1500				271	226	196	173	155
	1800					324	263	223	194
	2100							316	261
70	1200	Values in table are		244	211	187	169	154
	1500	time in days to		338	278	238	208	186
	1800	lose weight			325	272	235
	2100	indicated.				396	321
80	1200					251	221	199	181
	1500					336	284	247	219
	1800						397	327	280
	2100								389

Table A.29 Weight Loss Prediction: Men 56 - 75, 5' 6" - 5' 11" Activity Level 0

WEIGHT LOSS PREDICTION – MEN 56 to 75

Height: 5' 6" to 5' 11"   Activity Level 1

Weight Loss (lbs)	Diet Calories	Present Weight (lbs)							
		140	160	180	200	220	240	260	280
10	1200	39	33	28	25	22	20	19	17
	1500	57	44	37	31	27	24	22	20
	1800	102	68	51	41	35	30	27	24
	2100		145	86	62	48	40	34	30
20	1200		69	59	52	46	42	39	36
	1500		95	77	65	57	51	46	42
	1800		150	110	88	73	63	55	50
	2100		372	194	134	103	84	71	62
30	1200		109	92	81	72	65	59	55
	1500		152	122	102	89	78	70	64
	1800		253	179	140	115	98	86	77
	2100			340	220	165	132	111	96
40	1200			129	112	99	89	81	75
	1500			172	143	123	108	97	88
	1800			261	199	162	137	119	106
	2100				329	237	187	155	133
50	1200			168	145	128	115	104	96
	1500			229	188	160	140	124	112
	1800			364	267	213	179	154	136
	2100				323	249	204	173
60	1200				181	159	142	128	117
	1500				238	200	174	154	139
	1800				349	272	225	193	169
	2100					321	258	217
70	1200	Values in table are		221	192	170	154	140
	1500	time in days to		295	245	211	186	166
	1800	lose weight			341	277	235	205
	2100	indicated.				320	266
80	1200					228	201	181	164
	1500					295	251	220	196
	1800						336	281	243
	2100							393	321

Table A.30 Weight Loss Prediction: Men 56 - 75, 5' 6" - 5' 11" Activity Level 1

WEIGHT LOSS PREDICTION – MEN 56 to 75

Height: 5' 6" to 5' 11"   Activity Level 2

Weight Loss (lbs)	Diet Calories	Present Weight (lbs)							
		140	160	180	200	220	240	260	280
10	1200	32	27	23	21	19	17	15	14
	1500	43	34	29	25	22	20	18	16
	1800	65	47	37	31	27	23	21	19
	2100	133	75	53	41	34	29	25	22
20	1200		57	49	43	39	35	32	30
	1500		73	61	52	46	41	37	34
	1800		102	80	65	56	48	43	39
	2100		172	116	88	71	60	52	46
30	1200		89	76	67	60	54	49	46
	1500		117	96	81	71	63	57	52
	1800		168	127	103	87	75	67	60
	2100		305	191	141	113	94	81	71
40	1200			106	93	82	74	68	62
	1500			134	113	98	87	78	71
	1800			182	145	121	105	92	82
	2100			288	204	159	131	112	98
50	1200			139	120	106	95	87	80
	1500			178	148	127	112	100	91
	1800			248	193	159	136	119	106
	2100				280	213	173	146	127
60	1200				150	132	118	107	98
	1500				187	159	139	124	112
	1800				248	201	170	148	131
	2100				376	275	220	184	159
70	1200	Values in table are			182	159	142	128	117
	1500	time in days to			230	194	168	149	134
	1800	lose weight			314	249	208	179	158
	2100	indicated.				351	273	225	193
80	1200					189	167	150	137
	1500					233	200	176	158
	1800					304	250	214	187
	2100						336	272	230

Table A.31 Weight Loss Prediction: Men 56 - 75, 5' 6" - 5' 11" Activity Level 2

WEIGHT LOSS PREDICTION – MEN 56 to 75

Height: 5' 6" to 5' 11"   Activity Level 3

Weight Loss (lbs)	Diet Calories	Present Weight (lbs)							
		140	160	180	200	220	240	260	280
10	1200	25	21	18	16	15	13	12	11
	1500	31	25	22	19	17	15	14	12
	1800	41	32	26	22	19	17	15	14
	2100	61	43	33	27	23	20	17	16
20	1200		44	38	34	30	28	25	23
	1500		54	45	39	35	31	28	26
	1800		68	55	46	40	35	32	29
	2100		93	70	57	48	41	36	33
30	1200		70	60	53	47	43	39	36
	1500		85	71	61	54	48	44	40
	1800		110	88	73	63	55	49	45
	2100		155	114	90	75	64	57	50
40	1200			83	73	65	59	53	49
	1500			100	85	74	66	60	55
	1800			124	102	87	76	68	61
	2100			164	128	105	90	78	69
50	1200			109	94	84	75	69	63
	1500			131	111	96	85	77	70
	1800			166	134	114	99	87	79
	2100			226	171	138	117	101	90
60	1200				118	104	93	84	77
	1500				139	120	106	95	86
	1800				171	143	123	108	97
	2100				222	176	147	126	111
70	1200	Values in table are		143	125	112	101	92
	1500	time in days to		171	146	128	114	103
	1800	lose weight		213	175	150	131	117
	2100	indicated.		283	219	180	154	134
80	1200					149	132	119	108
	1500					175	152	135	121
	1800					212	179	155	138
	2100					270	218	184	159

Table A.32 Weight Loss Prediction: Men 56 - 75, 5' 6" - 5' 11" Activity Level 3

WEIGHT LOSS PREDICTION – MEN 56 to 75

Height: 6' 0" to 6' 6"   Activity Level 0

Weight Loss (lbs)	Diet Calories	Present Weight (lbs)							
		160	180	200	220	240	260	280	300
10	1200	32	28	25	22	20	19	17	16
	1500	43	36	31	27	24	22	20	19
	1800	65	50	41	35	30	27	24	22
	2100	132	82	60	48	40	34	30	27
20	1200		58	51	46	42	39	36	34
	1500		75	65	57	51	46	42	39
	1800		107	86	73	63	56	50	46
	2100		184	130	102	84	72	63	56
30	1200		91	80	72	65	60	55	51
	1500		119	101	88	78	71	65	59
	1800		172	137	114	98	87	78	70
	2100		316	213	163	132	112	97	86
40	1200			110	98	89	81	75	70
	1500			140	122	108	97	88	81
	1800			194	160	136	119	107	96
	2100			315	233	186	156	135	119
50	1200			143	127	114	104	96	89
	1500			184	158	139	125	113	104
	1800			259	210	178	155	137	124
	2100				315	247	204	175	153
60	1200				157	141	128	118	109
	1500				197	173	154	139	127
	1800				267	223	193	170	153
	2100					317	258	219	191
70	1200	Values in table are		189	169	153	141	130
	1500	time in days to		241	209	185	167	152
	1800	lose weight		332	274	234	205	184
	2100	indicated.				319	267	231
80	1200					200	180	165	152
	1500					249	219	196	178
	1800					331	280	243	216
	2100							321	275

Table A.33 Weight Loss Prediction: Men 56 to 75, 6' 0" to 6' 6", Activity Level 0

WEIGHT LOSS PREDICTION – MEN 56 to 75

Height: 6' 0" to 6' 6"   Activity Level 1

Weight Loss (lbs)	Diet Calories	Present Weight (lbs)							
		160	180	200	220	240	260	280	300
10	1200	29	26	23	20	19	17	16	15
	1500	38	32	28	24	22	20	18	17
	1800	55	43	36	30	27	24	21	20
	2100	96	65	49	41	34	29	26	23
20	1200		53	47	42	39	36	33	31
	1500		67	58	51	46	41	38	35
	1800		92	75	64	56	49	45	41
	2100		143	106	85	71	61	54	48
30	1200		83	73	66	60	55	51	47
	1500		106	90	79	71	64	58	54
	1800		147	118	100	87	77	69	63
	2100		239	171	135	112	96	84	75
40	1200			101	90	82	75	69	64
	1500			126	109	97	87	80	73
	1800			167	139	120	106	95	86
	2100			249	192	157	133	116	103
50	1200			131	116	105	96	88	82
	1500			164	142	125	112	102	94
	1800			222	183	156	136	122	110
	2100			345	257	207	174	150	133
60	1200				144	129	118	108	100
	1500				177	156	139	126	115
	1800				231	195	170	151	136
	2100				335	263	218	188	165
70	1200	Values in table are		174	155	141	129	119
	1500	time in days to		216	188	167	151	138
	1800	lose weight		286	239	206	182	163
	2100	indicated.			329	268	228	199
80	1200					183	165	151	139
	1500					223	197	177	161
	1800					287	245	215	192
	2100						325	273	236

Table A.34 Weight Loss Prediction: Men 56 to 75, 6' 0" to 6' 6", Activity Level 1

WEIGHT LOSS PREDICTION – MEN 56 to 75
Height: 6' 0" to 6' 6"   Activity Level 2

Weight Loss (lbs)	Diet Calories	Present Weight (lbs)							
		160	180	200	220	240	260	280	300
10	1200	25	21	19	17	16	14	13	12
	1500	31	26	23	20	18	16	15	14
	1800	40	33	28	24	21	19	17	16
	2100	59	44	35	29	25	22	20	18
20	1200		45	40	36	33	30	28	26
	1500		54	47	42	37	34	31	29
	1800		69	58	50	44	39	36	33
	2100		95	75	62	53	47	41	37
30	1200		70	62	55	50	46	43	40
	1500		86	74	65	58	52	48	44
	1800		110	91	78	68	61	55	50
	2100		155	119	98	83	72	64	58
40	1200			85	76	69	63	58	54
	1500			102	89	80	72	66	61
	1800			128	108	94	84	75	69
	2100			170	137	116	100	88	71
50	1200			110	98	88	81	74	69
	1500			133	116	103	92	84	77
	1800			168	141	122	108	97	88
	2100			230	182	151	130	114	102
60	1200				121	109	99	91	85
	1500				144	127	114	104	95
	1800				178	153	134	120	108
	2100				233	191	163	142	126
70	1200	Values in table are			146	131	119	109	101
	1500	time in days to			175	154	137	124	114
	1800	lose weight			219	186	162	144	130
	2100	indicated.			293	236	198	172	152
80	1200					154	140	128	118
	1500					182	162	146	133
	1800					222	192	170	153
	2100					287	238	205	180

Table A.35 Weight Loss Prediction: Men 56 to 75, 6' 0" to 6' 6", Activity Level 2

WEIGHT LOSS PREDICTION – MEN 56 to 75
Height: 6' 0" to 6' 6"   Activity Level 3

Weight Loss (lbs)	Diet Calories	Present Weight (lbs)							
		160	180	200	220	240	260	280	300
10	1200	20	17	15	14	13	11	11	10
	1500	23	20	17	15	14	13	12	11
	1800	29	24	20	18	16	14	13	12
	2100	37	29	24	21	18	16	15	13
20	1200		36	32	29	26	24	22	21
	1500		42	36	32	29	27	24	23
	1800		50	43	37	33	30	27	25
	2100		62	51	43	38	34	30	28
30	1200		56	49	44	40	37	34	32
	1500		65	57	50	45	41	38	35
	1800		79	67	58	51	46	42	38
	2100		100	81	68	59	52	47	43
40	1200			68	61	55	51	48	43
	1500			79	69	62	56	51	47
	1800			93	80	71	63	57	52
	2100			114	95	82	72	64	58
50	1200			88	79	71	65	60	55
	1500			102	90	80	72	66	61
	1800			122	104	91	81	73	67
	2100			151	125	107	93	83	75
60	1200				97	88	80	73	68
	1500				112	99	89	81	74
	1800				131	114	101	91	82
	2100				158	134	116	103	92
70	1200	Values in table are time in days to lose weight indicated.			117	105	95	87	81
	1500				135	119	107	97	89
	1800				160	138	121	109	99
	2100				195	163	141	124	111
80	1200					124	112	102	94
	1500					141	126	114	104
	1800					164	144	128	116
	2100					196	168	147	131

Table A.36 Weight Loss Prediction: Men 56 to 75, 6' 0" to 6' 6", Activity Level 3

Appendix B Weight Loss Prediction Tables - Women

This appendix contains 24 Weight Loss Prediction Tables for Women. The tables cover women from 18 to 75 years, with heights ranging from 4' 11" to 6' 0", and activity levels from 0 to 4. Refer to the index in Table BB below to find the table that's right for you.

Note, before choosing your personal Weight Loss Prediction table, you must determine your Activity Level. (See **Table 1** on page 17.)

Age	Height	Activity Levels	Tables on Pages
18 - 35	4' 11" to 5' 5"	1 to 4	90 to 93
18 - 35	5' 6" to 6' 0"	1 to 4	94 to 97
36 - 55	4' 11" to 5' 5"	0 to 3	98 to 101
36 - 55	5' 6" to 6' 0"	0 to 3	102 to 105
56 - 75	4' 11" to 5' 5"	0 to 3	106 to 109
56 - 75	5' 6" to 6' 0"	0 to 3	110 to 113

Table BB: 24 Weight Loss Prediction Tables for Women

Once you have selected the Weight Loss Prediction table that's appropriate for you, return to **Example 1** on page 35 for instruction on how to use the data in the table.

WEIGHT LOSS PREDICTION – WOMEN 18 to 35

Height: 4' 11" to 5' 5"   Activity Level 1

Weight Loss (lbs)	Diet Calories	Present Weight (lbs)							
		110	120	130	140	160	180	200	220
5	900	19	17	16	15	13	11	10	9
	1200	28	24	21	19	16	14	12	11
	1500	49	39	32	28	22	18	15	13
	1800	210	99	66	49	33	25	20	17
10	900	40	36	33	30	26	23	21	19
	1200	58	50	44	40	33	29	25	23
	1500	106	82	68	58	45	37	32	28
	1800		234	145	106	70	52	42	35
15	900		55	51	46	40	36	32	29
	1200		78	69	62	51	44	39	35
	1500		132	107	91	70	57	49	42
	1800			245	172	110	81	65	55
20	900		76	69	63	55	48	44	40
	1200		108	95	85	70	60	53	47
	1500		188	151	126	96	78	66	58
	1800			380	252	154	113	89	74
30	900			109	100	86	75	67	61
	1200			153	135	110	94	82	73
	1500			257	209	155	124	104	90
	1800				261	183	142	117	
40	900				140	119	104	92	84
	1200				193	155	130	113	100
	1500				315	223	175	145	124
	1800					267	203	164	
50	900	Values in table are		185	155	134	119	107	
	1200	time in days to		262	205	170	147	129	
	1500	lose weight			306	233	190	162	
	1800	indicated.				374	273	217	
60	900			237	195	168	148	133	
	1200			348	264	215	183	160	
	1500				302	242	203		
	1800					357	277		

Table B.1 Weight Loss Prediction Women 18 - 35 4' 11" - 5' 5" Activity Level 1

WEIGHT LOSS PREDICTION – WOMEN   18 to 35

Height: 4' 11" to 5' 5"   Activity Level 2

Weight Loss (lbs)	Diet Calories	Present Weight (lbs)							
		110	120	130	140	160	180	200	220
5	900	16	15	13	12	11	10	9	8
	1200	22	19	17	16	13	11	10	9
	1500	34	28	24	21	17	14	12	11
	1800	73	50	39	31	23	18	15	13
10	900	34	31	28	26	22	20	18	16
	1200	46	40	36	32	27	24	21	19
	1500	72	59	50	44	35	29	25	22
	1800	168	110	83	67	48	38	31	27
15	900		47	43	40	34	30	27	25
	1200		63	56	50	42	36	32	29
	1500		94	79	68	54	45	39	34
	1800		184	134	106	75	59	48	41
20	900		65	59	54	47	41	37	34
	1200		87	77	69	57	49	43	39
	1500		132	110	94	74	61	53	46
	1800		279	194	150	104	81	66	56
30	900			93	85	73	64	57	52
	1200			123	110	90	77	68	60
	1500			183	154	118	97	82	72
	1800			362	261	172	129	105	88
40	900				120	102	89	79	71
	1200				156	127	107	93	83
	1500				227	169	136	114	99
	1800					255	186	147	123
50	900	Values in table are time in days to lose weight indicated.			158	133	115	102	92
	1200				211	168	140	121	107
	1500				321	229	180	150	129
	1800					366	253	196	161
60	900				202	167	143	126	113
	1200				277	214	177	151	133
	1500					302	231	189	161
	1800						336	252	204

Table B.2   Weight Loss Prediction: Women 18 - 35, 4' 11" - 5' 5" Activity Level 2

WEIGHT LOSS PREDICTION – WOMEN   18 to 35

Height: 4' 11" to 5' 5"   Activity Level 3

Weight Loss (lbs)	Diet Calories	Present Weight (lbs)							
		110	120	130	140	160	180	200	220
5	900	13	12	11	10	9	8	7	6
	1200	17	15	13	12	10	9	8	7
	1500	23	19	17	15	12	10	9	8
	1800	36	28	23	20	15	13	11	9
10	900	27	25	23	21	18	16	14	13
	1200	35	31	28	25	21	18	16	15
	1500	48	41	36	31	26	22	19	17
	1800	78	60	49	42	32	26	22	19
15	900		38	35	32	28	25	22	20
	1200		48	43	39	33	28	25	23
	1500		64	55	49	40	33	29	26
	1800		97	78	66	50	41	34	30
20	900		53	48	44	38	34	30	27
	1200		66	59	53	45	39	34	31
	1500		90	77	67	54	46	40	35
	1800		139	110	92	69	56	47	41
30	900			76	69	59	52	47	42
	1200			95	85	70	60	53	48
	1500			126	109	86	72	62	54
	1800			189	153	112	89	74	63
40	900				97	83	72	64	58
	1200				120	99	84	73	65
	1500				158	122	101	86	75
	1800				231	162	125	103	88
50	900	Values in table are time in days to lose weight indicated.			128	108	93	83	74
	1200				161	130	110	95	84
	1500				218	164	133	112	97
	1800				343	222	168	136	115
60	900				164	136	117	103	92
	1200				210	165	138	119	105
	1500				295	213	169	141	121
	1800					301	218	173	144

Table B.3 Weight Loss Prediction: Women 18 - 35 4' 11" - 5' 5" Activity Level 3

WEIGHT LOSS PREDICTION – WOMEN 18 to 35
Height: 4' 11" to 5' 5"   Activity Level 4

Weight Loss (lbs)	Diet Calories	Present Weight (lbs)							
		110	120	130	140	160	180	200	220
5	900	10	9	8	8	7	6	5	5
	1200	12	11	10	9	8	7	6	5
	1500	14	13	11	10	9	7	7	6
	1800	19	16	14	12	10	8	7	6
10	900	20	19	17	16	14	12	11	10
	1200	24	22	20	18	15	13	12	11
	1500	29	26	23	21	17	15	13	12
	1800	38	33	28	25	20	17	15	13
15	900		29	26	24	21	19	17	15
	1200		34	30	28	24	21	18	16
	1500		41	36	32	27	23	20	18
	1800		51	44	39	31	26	22	20
20	900		39	36	33	28	25	23	20
	1200		46	41	38	32	28	25	22
	1500		56	49	44	36	31	27	24
	1800		72	61	53	42	35	31	27
30	900			56	51	44	39	35	31
	1200			66	59	50	43	38	34
	1500			79	70	57	49	42	38
	1800			100	86	67	56	48	42
40	900				72	61	54	48	43
	1200				84	70	60	53	47
	1500				100	81	68	58	52
	1800				125	96	78	66	57
50	900	Values in table are time in days to lose weight indicated.				80	69	61	55
	1200					91	78	68	60
	1500					107	89	76	67
	1800					128	103	86	74
60	900						86	76	68
	1200						97	84	75
	1500						112	95	83
	1800						131	108	93

Table B.4 Weight Loss Prediction Women 18 - 35 4' 11" - 5' 5" Activity Level 4

WEIGHT LOSS PREDICTION – WOMEN   18 to 35
Height: 5' 6" to 6' 0"   Activity Level 1

Weight Loss (lbs)	Diet Calories	Present Weight (lbs)							
		130	140	150	160	180	200	220	240
5	900	14	13	12	12	10	9	9	8
	1200	19	17	16	15	13	11	10	9
	1500	27	24	21	19	16	14	12	11
	1800	48	39	32	28	22	18	15	13
10	900	30	28	26	24	22	20	18	17
	1200	39	36	33	30	26	23	21	19
	1500	57	50	44	40	33	29	25	23
	1800	104	82	68	58	45	37	32	28
20	900		58	54	51	45	41	37	34
	1200		76	69	63	55	48	43	40
	1500		108	94	84	70	60	52	47
	1800		186	150	126	96	78	66	57
30	900			85	79	70	63	57	53
	1200			109	100	85	75	67	61
	1500			152	135	110	93	82	73
	1800			255	208	154	124	104	90
40	900				110	96	86	78	72
	1200				140	119	104	92	84
	1500				192	155	130	113	100
	1800				313	222	175	145	124
50	900					125	111	100	92
	1200					155	134	119	107
	1500					205	170	146	129
	1800					305	233	190	162
60	900	Values in table are				155	137	124	113
	1200	time in days to				195	168	148	132
	1500	lose weight				263	215	183	160
	1800	indicated.					301	241	203
70	900						166	149	135
	1200						204	178	159
	1500						265	223	194
	1800						383	300	248

Table B.5 Weight Loss Prediction Women 18 - 35, 5' 6" - 6' 0" Activity Level 1

WEIGHT LOSS PREDICTION – WOMEN 18 to 35

Height: 5' 6" to 6' 0"   Activity Level 2

Weight Loss (lbs)	Diet Calories	Present Weight (lbs)							
		130	140	150	160	180	200	220	240
5	900	12	12	11	10	9	8	7	7
	1200	16	14	13	12	11	9	8	8
	1500	21	19	17	15	13	11	10	9
	1800	32	27	23	20	16	14	12	10
10	900	26	24	22	21	19	17	15	14
	1200	33	30	27	25	22	19	18	16
	1500	44	39	35	32	27	23	20	18
	1800	68	56	48	42	34	28	25	22
20	900		50	47	44	39	35	32	29
	1200		63	57	53	46	41	37	33
	1500		84	74	67	56	48	43	38
	1800		124	105	91	72	60	51	45
30	900			73	68	60	54	49	45
	1200			91	83	72	63	56	51
	1500			119	106	88	7694	66	59
	1800			173	147	114		80	70
40	900				95	83	74	67	62
	1200				116	99	87	78	70
	1500				151	123	105	92	81
	1800				215	163	132	112	97
50	900					108	96	86	79
	1200					130	113	100	90
	1500					163	137	119	105
	1800					220	175	146	126
60	900	Values in table are time in days to lose weight indicated.				134	119	107	97
	1200					163	140	124	111
	1500					207	172	148	130
	1800					288	223	184	157
70	900						143	128	116
	1200						171	150	134
	1500						212	180	157
	1800						280	226	191

Table B.6 Weight Loss Prediction Women 18 - 35, 5' 6" - 6' 0" Activity Level 2

WEIGHT LOSS PREDICTION – WOMEN 18 to 35

Height: 5' 6" to 6' 0"   Activity Level 3

Weight Loss (lbs)	Diet Calories	Present Weight (lbs)							
		130	140	150	160	180	200	220	240
5	900	10	9	9	8	7	7	6	5
	1200	12	11	10	10	8	7	7	6
	1500	15	14	12	11	10	8	8	7
	1800	21	18	16	14	12	10	9	8
10	900	21	20	18	17	15	14	12	11
	1200	26	23	22	20	17	15	14	13
	1500	32	29	26	24	20	18	16	14
	1800	44	37	33	29	24	21	18	16
20	900		42	39	36	32	29	26	24
	1200		50	45	42	37	32	29	26
	1500		62	55	50	43	37	33	30
	1800		82	71	63	51	44	38	34
30	900			60	56	50	44	40	37
	1200			72	66	57	50	45	41
	1500			88	80	67	58	51	46
	1800			115	101	81	68	59	52
40	900				78	68	61	55	51
	1200				92	79	69	62	56
	1500				113	94	80	71	63
	1800				145	115	95	82	72
50	900					89	79	71	65
	1200					103	90	80	72
	1500					123	105	91	81
	1800					153	125	107	93
60	900	Values in table are time in days to lose weight indicated.				110	98	88	80
	1200					129	112	99	89
	1500					156	131	114	101
	1800					197	159	134	116
70	900						118	105	95
	1200						136	119	107
	1500						161	138	122
	1800						197	164	141

Table B.7 Weight Loss Prediction Women 18 - 35, 5' 6" - 6' 0" Activity Level 3

WEIGHT LOSS PREDICTION – WOMEN 18 to 35
Height: 5' 6" to 6' 0"   Activity Level 4

Weight Loss (lbs)	Diet Calories	Present Weight (lbs)							
		130	140	150	160	180	200	220	240
5	900	8	7	7	7	6	5	5	4
	1200	9	8	8	7	6	6	5	5
	1500	11	10	9	8	7	6	6	5
	1800	13	11	10	9	8	7	6	6
10	900	16	15	14	13	12	11	10	9
	1200	19	17	16	15	13	12	10	10
	1500	22	20	18	17	14	13	11	10
	1800	26	23	21	19	16	14	12	11
20	900		31	29	27	24	22	20	18
	1200		36	33	31	27	24	21	20
	1500		42	38	35	30	26	23	21
	1800		50	44	40	34	29	26	23
30	900			46	42	37	34	30	28
	1200			52	48	41	37	33	30
	1500			60	54	46	41	36	33
	1800			71	63	53	45	40	35
40	900				59	52	46	42	38
	1200				66	57	50	45	41
	1500				76	64	56	50	44
	1800				90	74	63	55	49
50	900					67	59	53	49
	1200					74	65	58	53
	1500					84	73	64	57
	1800					97	82	71	63
60	900	Values in table are time in days to lose weight indicated.				83	73	66	60
	1200					93	81	72	65
	1500					106	91	79	71
	1800					123	103	88	78
70	900						88	79	71
	1200						98	87	78
	1500						110	96	85
	1800						126	107	94

Table B.8 Weight Loss Prediction Women 18 - 35, 5' 6" - 6' 0" Activity Level 4

WEIGHT LOSS PREDICTION – WOMEN 36 to 55

Height: 4' 11" to 5' 5"   Activity Level 0

Weight Loss (lbs)	Diet Calories	Present Weight (lbs)							
		110	120	130	140	160	180	200	220
5	900	22	20	18	17	14	13	11	10
	1200	34	29	25	23	19	16	14	13
	1500	72	53	43	36	27	22	18	16
	1800		329	129	81	47	34	26	22
10	900	46	41	37	34	30	26	24	22
	1200	71	60	53	47	39	33	29	26
	1500	159	115	90	75	56	45	38	33
	1800			313	181	100	70	54	44
15	900		63	58	53	46	40	36	33
	1200		95	52	73	60	51	45	40
	1500		187	144	118	87	70	58	50
	1800				310	160	110	84	69
20	900		87	79	72	62	55	49	45
	1200		132	114	101	82	70	61	54
	1500		275	206	166	121	96	80	69
	1800					229	153	116	94
30	900			125	114	97	85	76	69
	1200			185	162	130	109	95	84
	1500			366	281	196	152	125	107
	1800						254	187	149
40	900				160	135	117	104	94
	1200				233	183	152	131	115
	1500					287	217	176	149
	1800						383	269	210
50	900	Values in table are time in days to lose weight indicated.			212	176	152	134	121
	1200				320	244	200	170	149
	1500						292	233	195
	1800							370	281
60	900				271	222	190	167	149
	1200					315	253	213	185
	1500						383	297	245
	1800								364

Table B.9 Weight Loss Prediction: Women 36-55, 4' 11"-5' 5" Activity Level 0

WEIGHT LOSS PREDICTION – WOMEN   36 to 55

Height: 4' 11" to 5' 5"   Activity Level 1

Weight Loss (lbs)	Diet Calories	Present Weight (lbs)							
		110	120	130	140	160	180	200	220
5	900	20	18	17	15	13	12	10	10
	1200	30	26	23	20	17	14	13	11
	1500	56	43	35	30	23	19	16	14
	1800		134	80	57	37	27	22	18
10	900	42	38	34	32	27	24	22	20
	1200	62	54	47	42	35	30	26	24
	1500	122	92	75	63	48	39	33	29
	1800		341	181	125	78	57	45	38
15	900		58	53	49	42	37	33	30
	1200		84	73	65	54	46	40	36
	1500		149	118	99	75	61	51	45
	1800			316	205	123	89	70	58
20	900		80	72	66	57	50	45	41
	1200		116	101	90	74	63	55	49
	1500		215	168	138	103	83	70	61
	1800				306	174	123	96	79
30	900			115	105	89	78	70	63
	1200			164	144	116	98	85	76
	1500			290	231	167	132	110	94
	1800					299	202	154	125
40	900				147	124	108	96	87
	1200				207	164	137	118	104
	1500				353	242	187	154	131
	1800						298	220	176
50	900	Values in table are			194	162	140	124	111
	1200	time in days to			282	218	179	154	135
	1500	lose weight				335	251	202	171
	1800	indicated.						299	234
60	900				249	204	175	154	137
	1200				377	281	227	192	168
	1500						326	258	215
	1800							395	300

Table B.10 Weight Loss Prediction Women 36-55, 4' 11"-5' 5" Activity Level 1

WEIGHT LOSS PREDICTION – WOMEN   36 to 55

Height: 4' 11" to 5' 5"   Activity Level 2

Weight Loss (lbs)	Diet Calories	Present Weight (lbs)							
		110	120	130	140	160	180	200	220
5	900	17	15	14	13	11	10	9	8
	1200	23	20	18	16	14	12	10	9
	1500	37	30	26	22	18	15	13	11
	1800	90	58	43	35	25	19	16	14
10	900	35	32	29	27	23	20	18	17
	1200	49	43	38	34	28	25	22	19
	1500	80	64	54	47	37	31	26	23
	1800	214	129	93	73	52	40	33	28
15	900		49	45	41	36	31	28	26
	1200		66	59	53	44	38	33	30
	1500		102	85	73	57	47	40	35
	1800		219	152	117	81	62	51	43
20	900		68	61	56	48	43	38	35
	1200		92	81	72	60	51	45	40
	1500		144	119	101	78	64	55	48
	1800		344	223	167	113	86	70	59
30	900			97	89	76	66	59	54
	1200			130	115	94	80	70	62
	1500			199	166	125	102	86	75
	1800				297	187	138	111	93
40	900				124	105	92	81	74
	1200				165	133	112	97	86
	1500				246	180	143	120	103
	1800					281	200	157	129
50	900	Values in table are time in days to lose weight indicated.			165	138	119	105	94
	1200				223	176	146	126	111
	1500				352	244	190	157	134
	1800					274	209	170
60	900				211	173	149	130	117
	1200				295	225	185	157	138
	1500					325	245	199	168
	1800						368	270	216

Table B.11 Weight Loss Prediction Women 36-55, 4' 11"-5' 5" Activity Level 2

WEIGHT LOSS PREDICTION – WOMEN 36 to 55

Height: 4' 11" to 5' 5"   Activity Level 3

Weight Loss (lbs)	Diet Calories	Present Weight (lbs)							
		110	120	130	140	160	180	200	220
5	900	14	12	11	10	9	8	7	6
	1200	17	15	14	12	11	9	8	7
	1500	24	21	18	16	13	11	9	8
	1800	40	31	25	21	16	13	11	10
10	900	28	26	23	22	19	16	15	13
	1200	37	32	29	26	22	19	17	15
	1500	52	43	37	33	27	23	19	17
	1800	87	66	53	45	34	27	23	20
15	900		40	36	33	29	25	23	21
	1200		50	45	40	34	29	26	23
	1500		68	58	51	41	35	30	26
	1800		106	84	70	53	42	36	31
20	900		54	49	45	39	34	31	28
	1200		69	61	55	46	40	35	31
	1500		95	81	71	57	47	41	36
	1800		153	119	98	73	58	49	42
30	900			78	72	61	54	48	43
	1200			99	88	73	62	55	49
	1500			133	115	90	75	64	56
	1800			206	164	118	93	77	66
40	900				100	85	74	66	59
	1200				125	102	87	76	67
	1500				167	128	105	89	77
	1800				251	171	132	108	91
50	900	Values in table are		133	111	96	85	76
	1200	time in days to		168	135	113	98	87
	1500	lose weight		231	172	138	116	100
	1800	indicated.		381	238	177	142	119
60	900				169	140	120	105	94
	1200				220	172	143	122	108
	1500				316	224	176	146	125
	1800					325	230	181	150

Table B.12 Weight Loss Prediction Women 36-55 4' 11"-5' 5" Activity Level 3

WEIGHT LOSS PREDICTION – WOMEN   36 to 55

Height: 5' 6" to 6' 0"   Activity Level 0

Weight Loss (lbs)	Diet Calories	Present Weight (lbs)							
		130	140	150	160	180	200	220	240
5	900	17	16	15	14	12	11	10	9
	1200	23	21	19	18	15	13	12	11
	1500	37	32	28	24	20	17	15	13
	1800	89	63	49	40	30	24	20	17
10	900	35	32	30	28	25	23	21	19
	1200	49	44	40	36	31	28	25	22
	1500	78	66	57	51	42	35	31	27
	1800	204	137	104	85	62	49	41	35
20	900		68	63	59	52	47	43	39
	1200		93	84	76	65	57	51	46
	1500		145	124	109	88	74	64	57
	1800		341	242	189	133	104	85	73
30	900			99	92	81	72	66	60
	1200			133	120	102	89	79	71
	1500			203	175	139	116	100	88
	1800				327	218	166	135	114
40	900				127	111	99	90	82
	1200				169	142	123	109	98
	1500				254	197	162	138	121
	1800					323	238	190	159
50	900					144	128	115	105
	1200					186	160	141	126
	1500					264	213	180	157
	1800						323	252	208
60	900	Values in table are time in days to lose weight indicated.					158	142	129
	1200						200	175	156
	1500						271	226	196
	1800							324	263
70	900						191	171	155
	1200						244	211	187
	1500						338	278	238
	1800								325

Table B.13 Weight Loss Prediction Women 36-55, 5' 6" - 6' 0" Activity Level 0

WEIGHT LOSS PREDICTION – WOMEN   36 to 55
Height: 5' 6" to 6' 0"   Activity Level 1

Weight Loss (lbs)	Diet Calories	Present Weight (lbs)							
		130	140	150	160	180	200	220	240
5	900	16	14	13	13	11	10	9	8
	1200	21	19	17	16	14	12	11	10
	1500	32	27	24	21	18	15	13	12
	1800	63	48	38	32	25	20	17	15
10	900	32	30	28	26	23	21	19	17
	1200	44	39	36	33	28	25	22	20
	1500	66	57	50	44	37	31	27	24
	1800	138	102	82	68	51	41	35	30
20	900		63	58	54	48	43	39	36
	1200		83	75	59	59	52	46	42
	1500		124	107	95	77	65	57	51
	1800		241	184	150	110	88	73	63
30	900			91	85	74	67	61	56
	1200			119	109	92	81	72	65
	1500			174	152	122	102	89	78
	1800			323	253	179	140	115	98
40	900				118	103	92	83	76
	1200				153	129	112	99	89
	1500				219	172	143	123	108
	1800				392	261	199	162	137
50	900					133	118	106	97
	1200					168	145	128	115
	1500					229	188	160	140
	1800					364	267	213	179
60	900	Values in table are time in days to lose weight indicated.				166	146	131	120
	1200					212	181	159	142
	1500					296	238	200	174
	1800						349	272	225
70	900						177	158	143
	1200						221	192	170
	1500						295	245	211
	1800							341	277

Table B.14 Weight Loss Prediction: Women 36-55, 5' 6"-6' 0" Activity Level 1

WEIGHT LOSS PREDICTION – WOMEN 36 to 55

Height: 5' 6" to 6' 0"   Activity Level 2

Weight Loss (lbs)	Diet Calories	Present Weight (lbs)							
		130	140	150	160	180	200	220	240
5	900	13	12	11	11	9	8	8	7
	1200	17	15	14	13	11	10	9	8
	1500	24	21	18	17	14	12	11	9
	1800	38	31	26	23	18	15	14	11
10	900	28	26	24	22	20	18	16	15
	1200	35	32	29	27	23	21	19	17
	1500	49	43	38	34	29	25	22	20
	1800	81	65	55	47	37	31	27	23
20	900		54	50	46	41	37	33	31
	1200		68	62	47	49	43	39	35
	1500		93	82	73	61	52	46	41
	1800		146	120	102	80	65	56	48
30	900			78	72	64	57	52	47
	1200			98	89	76	67	60	54
	1500			132	117	96	81	71	63
	1800			201	168	127	103	87	75
40	900				101	88	78	71	65
	1200				125	106	93	82	74
	1500				166	134	113	98	87
	1800				249	182	145	121	105
50	900					114	101	91	83
	1200					139	120	106	95
	1500					178	148	127	112
	1800					248	193	159	136
60	900	Values in table are time in days to lose weight indicated.				142	125	112	102
	1200					175	150	132	118
	1500					228	187	159	139
	1800					329	248	201	170
70	900						151	135	122
	1200						182	159	142
	1500						230	194	168
	1800						314	249	208

Table B.15 Weight Loss Prediction: Women 36-55, 5' 6"- 6' 0" Activity Level 2

WEIGHT LOSS PREDICTION – WOMEN 36 to 55

Height: 5' 6" to 6' 0"   Activity Level 3

Weight Loss (lbs)	Diet Calories	Present Weight (lbs)							
		130	140	150	160	180	200	220	240
5	900	11	10	9	9	8	7	6	6
	1200	13	12	11	10	9	8	7	6
	1500	17	15	13	12	10	9	8	7
	1800	23	20	17	15	12	11	9	8
10	900	22	21	19	18	16	14	13	12
	1200	27	25	23	21	18	16	15	13
	1500	35	31	28	25	22	19	17	15
	1800	49	41	36	32	26	22	19	17
20	900		44	41	38	33	30	27	25
	1200		53	48	44	38	34	30	28
	1500		67	60	54	45	39	35	31
	1800		90	78	68	55	46	40	35
30	900			63	59	52	46	42	38
	1200			76	70	60	53	47	43
	1500			95	85	71	61	54	48
	1800			127	110	88	73	63	55
40	900				82	72	64	58	53
	1200				98	83	73	65	59
	1500				121	100	85	74	66
	1800				159	124	102	87	76
50	900					93	83	74	67
	1200					109	94	84	75
	1500					131	111	96	85
	1800					166	134	114	99
60	900	Values in table are				116	102	91	83
	1200	time in days to				137	118	104	93
	1500	lose weight				167	139	120	106
	1800	indicated.				215	171	143	123
70	900						123	110	99
	1200						143	125	112
	1500						171	146	128
	1800						213	175	150

Table B.16 Weight Loss Prediction Women 36-55, 5' 6"-6' 0" Activity Level 3

WEIGHT LOSS PREDICTION – WOMEN   56 to 75

Height: 4' 11" to 5' 5"   Activity Level 0

Weight Loss (lbs)	Diet Calories	Present Weight (lbs)							
		110	120	130	140	160	180	200	220
5	900	24	22	20	18	15	14	12	11
	1200	39	33	29	25	21	18	15	14
	1500	101	69	52	42	31	25	20	18
	1800			292	127	61	40	30	24
10	900	50	45	41	37	32	28	25	23
	1200	83	69	60	53	43	36	32	28
	1500	234	151	112	90	65	51	42	36
	1800				304	131	85	63	51
15	900		69	63	57	49	43	39	35
	1200		109	93	82	66	56	48	43
	1500		252	181	143	101	79	65	55
	1800					213	134	98	78
20	900		95	86	78	67	59	52	47
	1200		152	129	113	91	76	66	58
	1500		385	263	202	140	108	89	76
	1800					313	188	136	107
30	900			136	124	105	91	81	73
	1200			212	182	144	119	103	90
	1500				354	230	174	140	118
	1800						319	221	171
40	900				174	146	126	111	100
	1200				266	204	167	143	125
	1500					343	249	198	165
	1800							325	244
50	900	Values in table are		232	191	164	144	129	
	1200	time in days to		369	274	220	186	162	
	1500	lose weight			339	263	216		
	1800	indicated.					329		
60	900				299	242	205	179	159
	1200					357	281	234	201
	1500							338	274
	1800								

Table B.17 Weight Loss Prediction Women 56-75, 4' 11"-5' 5" Activity Level 0

Height: 4' 11" to 5' 5"   Activity Level 1

Weight Loss (lbs)	Diet Calories	Present Weight (lbs)							
		110	120	130	140	160	180	200	220
5	900	22	20	18	16	14	12	11	10
	1200	34	29	25	22	18	16	14	12
	1500	72	53	42	35	26	21	18	15
	1800		311	122	77	45	32	25	20
10	900	46	41	37	34	29	26	23	21
	1200	71	60	52	46	38	32	28	25
	1500	161	114	89	73	55	44	37	32
	1800			297	172	95	67	51	42
15	900		63	57	52	45	39	35	32
	1200		94	82	72	59	50	43	39
	1500		187	142	116	85	67	56	48
	1800				295	152	104	80	65
20	900		87	78	72	61	54	48	43
	1200		132	113	99	80	68	59	52
	1500		275	204	163	117	93	77	66
	1800					218	145	110	89
30	900			125	113	95	83	74	67
	1200			185	160	127	107	92	81
	1500			365	277	191	148	121	103
	1800					390	241	177	141
40	900				159	133	115	102	92
	1200				232	180	149	128	112
	1500				281	211	170	143
	1800					364	256	199
50	900	Values in table are			211	175	150	132	118
	1200	time in days to			320	241	196	166	145
	1500	lose weight				395	284	225	187
	1800	indicated.						351	266
60	900				272	221	187	164	146
	1200					313	249	208	180
	1500						374	288	236
	1800								345

Table B.18 Weight Loss Prediction: Women 56-75, 4' 11"-5' 5" Activity Level 1

WEIGHT LOSS PREDICTION – WOMEN   56 to 75

Height: 4' 11" to 5' 5"   Activity Level 2

Weight Loss (lbs)	Diet Calories	Present Weight (lbs)							
		110	120	130	140	160	180	200	220
5	900	18	16	15	14	12	10	9	8
	1200	26	22	20	18	15	13	11	10
	1500	44	35	29	25	19	16	14	12
	1800	140	77	53	41	28	21	17	15
10	900	38	34	31	28	25	22	19	18
	1200	54	47	41	37	31	26	23	20
	1500	95	74	61	52	40	33	28	25
	1800	385	177	117	88	59	45	36	30
15	900		53	48	44	38	33	30	27
	1200		73	64	57	47	40	35	31
	1500		118	96	81	63	51	43	38
	1800		318	194	142	93	70	56	47
20	900		73	66	60	51	45	40	36
	1200		102	88	78	64	55	48	43
	1500		169	135	113	86	70	59	51
	1800			294	205	130	96	77	64
30	900			104	95	80	70	62	56
	1200			143	126	102	86	75	66
	1500			231	188	139	111	93	80
	1800				382	218	156	122	101
40	900				133	112	97	86	77
	1200				181	143	120	103	91
	1500				283	200	157	129	111
	1800					336	227	173	141
50	900	Values in table are		177	147	126	111	99
	1200	time in days to		246	191	157	134	118
	1500	lose weight			275	209	170	144
	1800	indicated.				315	233	187
60	900				227	185	157	138	123
	1200				328	245	199	168	146
	1500					370	270	216	181
	1800							304	238

Table B.19 Weight Loss Prediction Women 56-75, 4' 11"-5' 5" Activity Level 2

WEIGHT LOSS PREDICTION – WOMEN 56 to 75

Height: 4' 11" to 5' 5"   Activity Level 3

Weight Loss (lbs)	Diet Calories	Present Weight (lbs)							
		110	120	130	140	160	180	200	220
5	900	14	13	12	11	9	8	7	7
	1200	19	16	15	13	11	10	8	8
	1500	27	23	19	17	14	11	10	9
	1800	47	35	28	23	18	14	12	10
10	900	30	27	25	23	20	17	15	14
	1200	40	35	31	28	23	20	18	16
	1500	57	48	41	36	29	24	21	18
	1800	105	76	60	49	37	30	25	21
15	900		42	38	35	30	26	24	21
	1200		54	48	43	36	31	27	24
	1500		75	64	55	44	37	32	28
	1800		124	95	78	57	46	38	33
20	900		58	52	48	41	36	32	29
	1200		75	66	59	49	42	37	33
	1500		105	89	77	61	50	43	38
	1800		181	136	110	80	63	52	44
30	900			83	75	64	56	50	45
	1200			106	94	77	66	57	51
	1500			147	125	97	79	68	59
	1800			242	186	130	100	82	70
40	900				106	89	78	69	62
	1200				134	108	91	79	70
	1500				183	138	111	94	81
	1800				291	190	143	115	97
50	900	Values in table are time in days to lose weight indicated.			140	117	101	89	79
	1200				181	143	120	103	91
	1500				256	186	148	123	106
	1800					266	193	153	127
60	900				180	147	126	110	98
	1200				237	183	151	129	113
	1500				357	244	189	155	132
	1800					372	253	195	160

Table B.20 Weight Loss Prediction: Women 56-75, 4' 11"-5' 5" Activity Level 3

WEIGHT LOSS PREDICTION – WOMEN 56 to 75

Height: 5' 6" to 6' 0"   Activity Level 0

Weight Loss (lbs)	Diet Calories	Present Weight (lbs)							
		130	140	150	160	180	200	220	240
5	900	18	17	16	15	13	12	11	10
	1200	26	23	21	19	16	14	13	12
	1500	44	37	32	28	22	19	16	14
	1800	146	88	63	49	35	27	22	19
10	900	38	35	32	30	27	24	22	20
	1200	54	48	43	40	34	30	26	24
	1500	94	78	66	58	46	39	34	30
	1800	367	198	137	105	73	56	46	39
20	900		73	68	63	55	50	45	41
	1200		103	92	84	71	62	55	50
	1500		172	144	124	98	82	70	62
	1800			335	243	159	120	96	81
30	900			106	98	86	77	70	64
	1200			147	132	111	96	85	77
	1500			239	202	156	128	109	96
	1800					265	193	153	127
40	900				137	119	106	95	87
	1200				187	155	133	117	105
	1500				297	223	180	152	132
	1800						279	217	178
50	900					154	136	123	112
	1200					204	173	152	135
	1500					301	238	199	171
	1800						385	290	234
60	900	Values in table are time in days to lose weight indicated.				193	169	151	137
	1200					258	217	189	167
	1500					396	305	251	214
	1800							376	298
70	900						205	182	164
	1200						266	229	202
	1500						383	309	261
	1800								371

Table B.21 Weight Loss Prediction Women 56-75, 5' 6"-6' 0" Activity Level 0

WEIGHT LOSS PREDICTION – WOMEN   56 to 75

Height: 5' 6" to 6' 0"   Activity Level 1

Weight Loss (lbs)	Diet Calories	Present Weight (lbs)							
		130	140	150	160	180	200	220	240
5	900	17	15	14	13	12	11	10	9
	1200	23	21	19	17	15	13	12	10
	1500	37	31	27	24	19	16	14	13
	1800	86	61	47	38	28	22	19	16
10	900	35	32	30	28	25	22	20	18
	1200	48	43	39	36	30	27	24	22
	1500	77	65	56	49	40	34	30	26
	1800	197	132	100	81	59	46	39	33
20	900		67	62	58	51	47	41	38
	1200		92	82	75	64	56	50	45
	1500		143	122	106	85	71	62	54
	1800		330	233	182	127	99	81	69
30	900			98	90	79	71	64	59
	1200			131	118	100	87	77	69
	1500			199	172	135	112	96	84
	1800				314	209	158	128	108
40	900				126	109	97	88	80
	1200				167	139	120	106	95
	1500				249	192	157	133	116
	1800					310	227	181	151
50	900					142	125	113	103
	1200					183	156	137	122
	1500					257	207	174	151
	1800						308	240	198
60	900	Values in table are				177	156	139	126
	1200	time in days to				231	195	170	151
	1500	lose weight				335	263	219	188
	1800	indicated.						309	250
70	900						188	167	151
	1200						239	206	182
	1500						329	269	229
	1800							390	310

Table B.22 Weight Loss Prediction: Women 56-75, 5' 6"-6' 0" Activity Level 1

WEIGHT LOSS PREDICTION – WOMEN   56 to 75

Height: 5' 6" to 6' 0"   Activity Level 2

Weight Loss (lbs)	Diet Calories	Present Weight (lbs)							
		130	140	150	160	180	200	220	240
5	900	14	13	12	11	10	9	8	7
	1200	18	17	15	14	12	11	9	9
	1500	26	23	20	18	15	13	11	10
	1800	45	36	30	25	20	16	14	12
10	900	29	27	25	23	21	19	17	15
	1200	38	35	31	29	25	22	20	18
	1500	55	48	42	37	31	27	23	21
	1800	97	76	63	53	41	34	29	25
20	900		57	53	49	43	39	35	32
	1200		74	67	61	52	46	41	37
	1500		103	90	80	65	56	49	43
	1800		174	139	116	88	71	60	52
30	900			83	77	67	60	54	50
	1200			105	96	81	71	63	57
	1500			146	128	103	87	76	67
	1800			237	193	142	113	94	81
40	900				107	93	82	74	68
	1200				135	113	98	87	78
	1500				184	146	122	105	92
	1800				291	205	160	132	112
50	900					120	106	95	87
	1200					148	128	112	100
	1500					194	160	136	119
	1800					281	214	173	147
60	900	Values in table are				150	132	118	107
	1200	time in days to				187	160	139	124
	1500	lose weight				250	202	171	148
	1800	indicated.				379	277	220	184
70	900						160	142	128
	1200						195	169	150
	1500						250	209	180
	1800						353	274	226

Table B.23 Weight Loss Prediction: Women 56-75, 5' 6"-6' 0" Activity Level 2

WEIGHT LOSS PREDICTION – WOMEN 56 to 75

Height: 5' 6" to 6' 0"   Activity Level 3

Weight Loss (lbs)	Diet Calories	Present Weight (lbs)							
		130	140	150	160	180	200	220	240
5	900	11	10	10	9	8	7	6	6
	1200	14	13	12	11	9	8	7	7
	1500	18	16	14	13	11	9	8	8
	1800	26	22	19	16	13	11	10	9
10	900	24	22	20	19	17	15	14	12
	1200	29	26	24	22	19	17	15	14
	1500	38	33	30	27	23	20	17	16
	1800	54	45	39	34	28	23	20	18
20	900		46	42	40	35	31	28	26
	1200		56	51	47	40	36	32	29
	1500		72	64	57	48	41	36	32
	1800		100	85	74	59	49	42	37
30	900			67	62	54	48	44	40
	1200			81	74	63	55	49	44
	1500			102	91	76	65	57	50
	1800			140	120	94	78	66	58
40	900				86	75	66	60	54
	1200				103	88	76	68	61
	1500				130	106	90	78	69
	1800				175	134	109	92	80
50	900					97	86	77	70
	1200					115	99	88	79
	1500					140	117	101	90
	1800					180	144	121	104
60	900	Values in table are time in days to lose weight indicated.				121	106	95	86
	1200					144	124	109	97
	1500					178	148	127	111
	1800					235	184	152	130
70	900						129	114	103
	1200						151	131	117
	1500						182	154	134
	1800						230	187	159

Table B.24 Weight Loss Prediction Women 56-75, 5' 6"-6' 0" Activity Level 3

Appendix C Weight Maintenance Tables - Men

This appendix contains nine Weight Maintenance Calorie Tables for Men. The tables cover men from 18 to 75 years, with heights ranging from 5' 0" to 6' 6", and activity levels from 0 to 4. Refer to the index shown in Table CC below to find the table that's right for you. Before choosing your personal Weight Maintenance Calorie table, you must determine your Activity Level (see **Table 1** on page 17).

Age	Height	Activity Levels	Tables On page
18 - 35	5' 0" to 5' 5"	1 to 4	115
18 - 35	5' 6" to 5' 11"	1 to 4	116
18 - 35	6' 0" to 6' 6"	1 to 4	117
36 - 55	5' 0" to 5' 5"	0 to 3	118
36 - 55	5' 6" to 5' 11"	0 to 3	119
36 - 55	6' 0" to 6' 6"	0 to 3	120
56 - 75	5' 0" to 5' 5"	0 to 3	121
56 - 75	5' 6" to 5' 11"	0 to 3	122
56 - 75	6' 0" to 6' 6"	0 to 3	123

Table CC: 9 Weight Maintenance Calorie Tables for Men

Once you have selected the Weight Maintenance Calorie table that's appropriate for you, return to **Example 2** on page 42 for instruction on how to use the data in the table.

WEIGHT MAINTENANCE CALORIES - MEN

Age: 18 to 35 yrs   Height: 5' 0" to 5' 5"

Weight (lbs)	ACTIVITY				
	Level 0	Level 1	Level 2	Level 3	Level 4
100	1853	1922	2080	2327	2797
105	1904	1976	2142	2402	2895
110	1954	2030	2203	2475	2992
115	2003	2082	2264	2548	3088
120	2051	2134	2323	2620	3184
125	2099	2185	2383	2691	3279
130	2146	2236	2441	2762	3373
135	2192	2285	2499	2832	3467
140	2238	2335	2556	2902	3560
150	2328	2432	2669	3040	3745
160	2416	2527	2780	3175	3927
170	2503	2621	2890	3309	4108
180	2588	2713	2997	3442	4288
190	2672	2804	3104	3573	4466
200	2754	2893	3209	3703	4643
210	2835	2981	3313	3832	4819
220	2916	3069	3416	3960	4994
230	2995	3155	3518	4086	5167
240	3073	3240	3619	4212	5340
250	3150	3324	3719	4337	5512
260	3227	3407	3818	4460	5682

Values in table are Calories per day.

Table C.1 Maintenance Calories: Men 18 - 35, 5' 0" to 5' 5"

WEIGHT MAINTENANCE CALORIES - MEN

Age: 18 to 35 yrs   Height: 5' 6" to 5' 11"

Weight (lbs)	ACTIVITY				
	Level 0	Level 1	Level 2	Level 3	Level 4
120	2160	2245	2434	2731	3295
125	2210	2298	2495	2804	3392
130	2259	2350	2556	2877	3488
135	2307	2402	2615	2949	3583
140	2355	2453	2674	3020	3678
145	2402	2504	2733	3091	3773
150	2448	2554	2791	3161	3866
155	2494	2604	2848	3231	3960
160	2540	2653	2905	3301	4053
170	2630	2750	3018	3438	4237
180	2718	2845	3129	3574	4420
190	2805	2939	3239	3708	4601
200	2890	3031	3347	3841	4781
210	2974	3122	3454	3973	4960
220	3057	3212	3560	4103	5137
230	3139	3301	3664	4232	5313
240	3220	3389	3768	4361	5489
250	3300	3476	3871	4488	5663
260	3378	3562	3972	4615	5837
270	3457	3647	4073	4740	6009
280	3534	3731	4173	4865	6181

Values in table are Calories per day.

Table C.2 Maintenance Calories: Men 18 - 35, 5' 6" to 5' 11"

WEIGHT MAINTENANCE CALORIES - MEN

Age: 18 to 35 yrs   Height: 6' 0" to 6' 6"

Weight (lbs)	ACTIVITY				
	Level 0	Level 1	Level 2	Level 3	Level 4
140	2453	2551	2772	3118	3776
145	2502	2603	2832	3191	3872
150	2550	2655	2892	3262	3967
155	2598	2706	2951	3334	4062
160	2645	2756	3009	3404	4156
165	2691	2806	3067	3475	4250
170	2737	2856	3125	3545	4344
175	2783	2905	3182	3614	4436
180	2828	2954	3238	3683	4529
190	2917	3050	3350	3820	4713
200	3005	3145	3461	3955	4895
210	3092	3239	3570	4089	5076
220	3177	3331	3678	4222	5256
230	3261	3422	3785	4353	5434
240	3344	3512	3891	4484	5612
250	3426	3601	3996	4613	5788
260	3507	3689	4100	4742	5964
270	3587	3776	4203	4870	6139
280	3667	3863	4305	4997	6313
290	3745	3948	4406	5123	6486
300	3823	4033	4507	5248	6658

Values in table are Calories per day.

Table C.3 Maintenance Calories: Men 18 - 35, 6' 0" to 6' 6"

WEIGHT MAINTENANCE CALORIES - MEN

Age: 36 to 55 yrs   Height: 5' 0" to 5' 5"

Weight (lbs)	ACTIVITY			
	Level 0	Level 1	Level 2	Level 3
100	1771	1841	1999	2246
105	1820	1893	2059	2318
110	1868	1945	2119	2390
115	1915	1996	2177	2461
120	1962	2046	2236	2532
125	2008	2096	2293	2602
130	2054	2145	2350	2671
135	2098	2193	2406	2740
140	2143	2241	2462	2808
150	2230	2335	2572	2943
160	2316	2428	2681	3076
170	2400	2519	2788	3207
180	2483	2609	2893	3338
190	2564	2697	2997	3466
200	2644	2784	3100	3594
210	2723	2870	3202	3720
220	2801	2955	3302	3846
230	2878	3039	3402	3970
240	2954	3122	3501	4094
250	3029	3204	3599	4216
260	3103	3285	3696	4338

Values in table are Calories per day.

Table C.4 Maintenance Calories: Men 36 - 55, 5' 0" to 5' 5"

WEIGHT MAINTENANCE CALORIES - MEN

Age: 36 to 55 yrs   Height: 5' 6" to 5' 11"

Weight (lbs)	ACTIVITY			
	Level 0	Level 1	Level 2	Level 3
120	2031	2115	2304	2601
125	2078	2166	2363	2672
130	2125	2216	2421	2742
135	2171	2265	2479	2812
140	2216	2314	2536	2881
145	2261	2363	2592	2950
150	2306	2411	2648	3018
155	2350	2459	2703	3086
160	2394	2506	2759	3154
170	2480	2599	2867	3287
180	2564	2690	2975	3419
190	2648	2781	3081	3550
200	2729	2869	3185	3679
210	2810	2957	3289	3808
220	2890	3044	3391	3935
230	2968	3129	3493	4061
240	3046	3214	3593	4186
250	3123	3298	3692	4310
260	3199	3381	3792	4434
270	3274	3463	3890	4557
280	3349	3545	3987	4679

Values in table are Calories per day.

Table C.5 Maintenance Calories: Men 36 - 55, 5' 6" to 5' 11"

WEIGHT MAINTENANCE CALORIES - MEN

Age: 36 to 55 yrs   Height: 6' 0" to 6' 6"

Weight (lbs)	ACTIVITY			
	Level 0	Level 1	Level 2	Level 3
140	2355	2453	2674	3020
145	2402	2504	2733	3091
150	2449	2554	2791	3161
155	2495	2604	2848	3231
160	2541	2653	2905	3301
165	2586	2701	2962	3370
170	2631	2750	3018	3438
175	2675	2797	3074	3506
180	2719	2845	3129	3574
190	2806	2939	3239	3708
200	2891	3031	3347	3841
210	2975	3122	3454	3973
220	3058	3212	3560	4103
230	3140	3301	3664	4232
240	3221	3389	3768	4361
250	3301	3476	3871	4488
260	3380	3562	3972	4615
270	3458	3647	4073	4740
280	3535	3731	4173	4865
290	3612	3815	4273	4989
300	3687	3897	4371	5112

Values in table are Calories per day.

Table C.6 Maintenance Calories: Men 36 - 55, 6' 0" to 6' 6"

WEIGHT MAINTENANCE CALORIES - MEN

Age: 56 to 75 yrs   Height: 5' 0" to 5' 5"

Weight (lbs)	ACTIVITY			
	Level 0	Level 1	Level 2	Level 3
100	1682	1752	1910	2157
105	1729	1803	1969	228
110	1776	1853	2026	2298
115	1821	1902	2083	2368
120	1866	1950	2140	2436
125	1911	1998	2196	2504
130	1955	2046	2251	2572
135	1998	2092	2306	2639
140	2041	2139	2360	2706
150	2125	2230	2467	2838
160	2208	2320	2573	2968
170	2289	2408	2677	3097
180	2369	2495	2779	3224
190	2448	2581	2881	3350
200	2525	2665	2981	3475
210	2602	2749	3080	3599
220	2677	2831	3179	3722
230	2752	2913	3276	3844
240	2825	2993	3373	3965
250	2898	3073	3468	4086
260	2970	3152	3563	4205

Values in table are Calories per day.

Table C.7 Maintenance Calories: Men 56 - 75, 5' 0" to 5' 5"

WEIGHT MAINTENANCE CALORIES - MEN

Age: 56 to 75 yrs   Height: 5' 6" to 5' 11"

Weight (lbs)	ACTIVITY			
	Level 0	Level 1	Level 2	Level 3
120	1927	2011	2201	2497
125	1973	2060	2258	2567
130	2018	2109	2314	2635
135	2062	2157	2370	2704
140	2106	2204	2425	2771
145	2150	2251	2480	2838
150	2192	2297	2534	2905
155	2235	2343	2588	2971
160	2277	2389	2642	3037
170	2360	2479	2748	3168
180	2442	2568	2852	3297
190	2522	2655	2955	3425
200	2601	2741	3057	3551
210	2679	2826	3158	3677
220	2756	2910	3258	3801
230	2832	2993	3357	3925
240	2907	3075	3455	4047
250	2982	3157	3552	4169
260	3055	3237	3648	4290
270	3128	3317	3744	4411
280	3201	3397	3839	4531

Values in table are Calories per day.

Table C.8 Maintenance Calories: Men 56 - 75, 5' 6" to 5' 11"

WEIGHT MAINTENANCE CALORIES - MEN

Age: 56 to 75 yrs   Height: 6' 0" to 6' 6"

Weight (lbs)	ACTIVITY			
	Level 0	Level 1	Level 2	Level 3
140	2237	2335	2556	2902
145	2282	2384	2613	2971
150	2327	2432	2669	3040
155	2371	2480	2725	3108
160	2415	2527	2780	3175
165	2459	2574	2835	3243
170	2502	2621	2890	3309
175	2545	2667	2944	3376
180	2587	2713	2997	3442
190	2671	2804	3104	3573
200	2753	2893	3209	3703
210	2834	2981	3313	3832
220	2915	3069	3416	3960
230	2994	3155	3518	4086
240	3072	3240	3619	4212
250	3149	3324	3719	4337
260	3225	3407	3817	4460
270	3301	3490	3917	4584
280	3376	3572	4014	4706
290	3450	3653	4111	4828
300	3524	3734	4208	4949

Values in table are Calories per day.

Table C.9 Maintenance Calories: Men 56 - 75 yrs, 6' 0" to 6' 6"

Appendix D Weight Maintenance Tables for Women

This appendix contains six Weight Maintenance Calorie Tables for Women. The tables cover women from 18 to 75 years, with heights ranging from 4' 11" to 6' 0", and activity levels from 0 to 4. Refer to the index shown in Table BB below to find the table that's right for you.

Before choosing your personal Weight Maintenance Calorie table, you must determine your Activity Level. (See **Table 1** on page 17.)

Age	Height	Activity Levels	Table No.
18 - 35	4' 11" to 5' 5"	1 to 4	**125**
18 - 35	5' 6" to 6' 0"	1 to 4	**126**
36 - 55	4' 11" to 5' 5"	0 to 3	**127**
36 - 55	5' 6" to 6' 0"	0 to 3	**128**
56 - 75	4' 11" to 5' 5"	0 to 3	**129**
56 - 75	5' 6" to 6' 0"	0 to 3	**130**

Table DD: 6 Weight Maintenance Calorie Tables for Women

Once you have selected the Weight Maintenance Calorie table that's appropriate for you, return to **Example 2** on page 42 for instruction on how to use the data in the table.

WEIGHT MAINTENANCE CALORIES - WOMEN

Age: 18 to 35 yrs   Height: 4' 11" to 5' 5"

Weight (lbs)	ACTIVITY				
	Level 0	Level 1	Level 2	Level 3	Level 4
100	1729	1799	1956	2204	2677
105	1777	1851	2016	2276	2772
110	1824	1901	2074	2347	2867
115	1870	1951	2132	2417	2961
120	1916	2001	2190	2487	3054
125	1962	2050	2246	2556	3147
130	2006	2098	2302	2624	3239
135	2050	2145	2358	2692	3331
140	2094	2193	2413	2759	3422
145	2137	2239	2467	2826	3512
150	2180	2286	2522	2893	3602
160	2264	2377	2629	3025	3781
170	2347	2467	2734	3155	3959
180	2428	2555	2838	3284	4135
190	2508	2642	2941	3411	4310
200	2587	2728	3042	3537	4483
210	2665	2813	3143	3663	4656
220	2741	2896	3242	3787	4827
230	2817	2979	3341	3910	4998
240	2892	3061	3439	4033	5168
250	2966	3142	3535	4154	5337

Values in table are Calories per day.

Table D.1 Maintenance Calories: Women 18 - 35, 4' 11" - 5' 5"

WEIGHT MAINTENANCE CALORIES - WOMEN

Age: 18 to 35 yrs   Height: 5' 6" to 6' 0"

Weight (lbs)	ACTIVITY				
	Level 0	Level 1	Level 2	Level 3	Level 4
100	1820	1890	2048	2295	2770
105	1870	1944	2110	2369	2868
110	1919	1996	2170	2442	2964
115	1968	2048	2230	2514	3060
120	2015	2099	2289	2585	3155
125	2062	2150	2347	2656	3250
130	2109	2200	2405	2726	3343
135	2155	2249	2463	2796	3437
140	2200	2298	2519	2865	3529
145	2245	2346	2575	2934	3622
150	2289	2394	2631	3002	3713
160	2376	2488	2741	3136	3895
170	2462	2581	2850	3270	4076
180	2546	2672	2957	3401	4255
190	2629	2762	3062	3531	4433
200	2710	2850	3166	3660	4609
210	2791	2938	3270	3788	4784
220	2870	3024	3372	3915	4958
230	2948	3109	3473	4041	5131
240	3026	3194	3573	4166	5303
250	3102	3277	3672	4290	5475

Values in table are Calories per day.

Table D.2 Maintenance Calories: Women 18 - 35, 5' 6" - 6' 0"

WEIGHT MAINTENANCE CALORIES - WOMEN

Age: 36 to 55 yrs   Height: 4' 11" to 5' 5"

Weight (lbs)	ACTIVITY			
	Level 0	Level 1	Level 2	Level 3
100	1682	1752	1910	2157
105	1729	1803	1969	2228
110	1776	1853	2026	2298
115	1821	1902	2083	2368
120	1866	1950	2140	2436
125	1911	1998	2196	2504
130	1955	2046	2251	2572
135	1998	2092	2306	2639
140	2041	2139	2360	2706
145	2083	2185	2414	2772
150	2125	2230	2467	2838
160	2208	2320	2573	2968
170	2289	2408	2677	3097
180	2369	2495	2779	3224
190	2448	2581	2881	3350
200	2525	2665	2981	3475
210	2602	2749	3080	3599
220	2677	2831	3179	3722
230	2752	2913	3276	3844
240	2825	2993	3373	3965
250	2898	3073	3468	4086

Values in table are Calories per day.

Table D.3 Maintenance Calories: Women 36 - 55, 4' 11" - 5' 5"

WEIGHT MAINTENANCE CALORIES - WOMEN

Age: 36 to 55 yrs   Height: 5' 6" to 6' 0"

Weight (lbs)	ACTIVITY			
	Level 0	Level 1	Level 2	Level 3
100	1739	1809	1967	2214
105	1787	1861	2027	2286
110	1835	1912	2085	2357
115	1881	1962	2144	2428
120	1927	2011	2201	2497
125	1973	2060	2258	2567
130	2018	2109	2314	2635
135	2062	2157	2370	2704
140	2106	2204	2425	2771
145	2150	2251	2480	2838
150	2192	2297	2534	2905
160	2277	2389	2642	3037
170	2360	2479	2748	3168
180	2442	2568	2852	3297
190	2522	2655	2955	3425
200	2601	2741	3057	3551
210	2679	2826	3158	3677
220	2756	2910	3258	3801
230	2832	2993	3357	3925
240	2907	3075	3455	4047
250	2982	3157	3552	4169

Values in table are Calories per day.

Table D.4 Maintenance Calories: Women 36 - 55, 5' 6" - 6' 0"

WEIGHT MAINTENANCE CALORIES - WOMEN

Age: 56 to 75 yrs   Height: 4' 11" to 5' 5"

Weight (lbs)	ACTIVITY			
	Level 0	Level 1	Level 2	Level 3
100	1608	1678	1836	2083
105	1653	1727	1893	2152
110	1698	1775	1949	2221
115	1742	1823	2005	2289
120	1786	1870	2060	2356
125	1829	1916	2114	2423
130	1871	1962	2168	2489
135	1913	2008	2221	2555
140	1955	2053	2274	2620
145	1996	2098	2327	2685
150	2037	2142	2379	2749
160	2117	2229	2482	2877
170	2196	2315	2584	3003
180	2274	2400	2684	3129
190	2350	2483	2783	3252
200	2425	2565	2881	3375
210	2500	2647	2978	3497
220	2573	2727	3075	3618
230	2646	2807	3170	3738
240	2717	2885	3265	3857
250	2789	2964	3359	3976

Values in table are Calories per day.

Table D.5 Maintenance Calories: Women 56 - 75, 4' 11" - 5' 5"

WEIGHT MAINTENANCE CALORIES - WOMEN

Age: 56 to 75 yrs   Height: 5' 6" to 6' 0"

Weight (lbs)	ACTIVITY			
	Level 0	Level 1	Level 2	Level 3
100	1665	1735	1893	2140
105	1711	1785	1951	2210
110	1757	1834	2008	2280
115	1803	1883	2065	2349
120	1847	1931	2121	2417
125	1891	1979	2176	2485
130	1935	2026	2231	2552
135	1978	2072	2286	2619
140	2020	2118	2340	2685
145	2062	2164	2393	2751
150	2104	2209	2446	2817
160	2186	2298	2551	2946
170	2267	2386	2655	3074
180	2346	2472	2757	3201
190	2424	2557	2858	3327
200	2501	2641	2957	3451
210	2577	2724	3056	3575
220	2652	2806	3154	3697
230	2726	2887	3251	3819
240	2800	2968	3347	3940
250	2872	3047	3442	4060

Values in table are Calories per day.

Table D.6 Maintenance Calories: Women 56 - 75, 5' 6" - 6' 0"

Appendix E Updated Weight Loss Model

At the time that Antonetti's weight-loss model was developed, the basil metabolic rate or the energy required to maintain the human body at rest was believed to best be represented by presuming it was dependent on body surface area [3]. But this assumption made the resulting weight loss predictive differential equation non-linear that required a relatively complex numerical solution using programmed software [4].

Then in 2016, professor Diana Thomas suggested the Antonetti model be updated by replacing the resting metabolic rate portion of the model with the much newer, validated and widely used Mifflin-St. Jeor regression equations [5]. As a bonus the update also eliminated the non-linearity in the Antonetti's original model and resulted in a differential equation with a much simpler closed-form solution, now called the Antonetti-Thomas weight loss model [6]. The most important advantage of the new Antonetti-Thomas model is that its solution is a relatively simple equation that can be used to directly solve practical weight loss prediction situations. (In fact, high-school algebra is all that is needed to use the Antonetti-Thomas model.) Before the new Antonetti-Thomas model is presented, however, some additional background is needed.

Physical Activity Energy (PA): This parameter has been shown to be directly proportional to an individual's weight. In other words for a given activity the more one weighs the more calories are burned. Expressed mathematically, $PA = KaW$, where Ka is the activity level coefficient and W is an individual's weight. Table 1 was adapted from [11]. The equivalent pedometer steps have been added by this writer.

Lifestyle	Ka (kcal/kg/d)	Approximate Daily Pedometer Steps
Sedentary	8	5000 or less
Light	10	About 6500
Moderate	13	About 8000
Vigorous	18	About 11500
Severe	27	17000 or more

Table 1: Activity Coefficient (Ka)

Resting Energy Expenditure: From Mifflin-St Jeor [5]:

For females: $B = 6.25H - 4.92A - 161$ For males: $B = 6.25H - 4.92A + 5$

where H is height (cm) and A is age (years). Two parameters that appear in the Antonetti-Thomas model are K_1 and K_2 which are defined as follows:

$K_1 = 0.9DI - B$ and $K_2 = Ka + 9.99$, where DI is dietary intake (kcal).

The derivation of the updated Antonetti-Thomas weight loss model is not covered here. (If interested in the details see Appendix F - Bibliography reference 6.) The Antonetti-Thomas model can be rearranged into three different versions to address the following types of problems:

1) Time to Lose Weight: How long will it take an individual to lose (or gain) a certain amount of weight. Solve for time:

$$t = -\frac{\gamma}{K_2} \ln\left[\frac{K_1 - K_2W_f}{K_1 - K_2W_0} \right] \qquad (1)$$

where t time on diet (days)

       γ energy value per unit of body mass lost = 7700 kcal/kg

       W_0 initial weight (kg)

       W_f final weight (kg)

2) Required Dietary Intake: What must the dietary intake of an individual be in order to lose (or gain) a certain amount of weight in a given amount of time? To solve for dietary intake use:

$$DI = \frac{(-K_2W_0 - B)\exp\left(-\frac{tK_2}{\gamma}\right) + K_2W_f + B}{\left(\exp\left(-\frac{tK_2}{\gamma}\right) - 1\right)(-1 + \alpha)} \qquad (2)$$

where α specific dynamic action of food $= 0.10$

The Weight Loss Model is continued on the next page.

3) Amount of Weight Lost:

3) Amount of Weight Lost: And still another way of thinking about the problem is: How much weight will an individual lose (or gain) on a specified dietary intake in a given amount of time? To solve this type of problem use the following version of the Antonetti-Thomas model:

$$W_f = \frac{(K_2 W_0 - K_1)\exp\left(-\dfrac{tK_2}{\gamma}\right) + K_1}{K_2} \qquad (3)$$

$$\Delta W = W_0 - W_f \qquad (4)$$

PRACTICAL EXAMPLES

The following examples illustrate the use of the different versions of the Antonetti-Thomas model.

Example 1. How long will it take a 30 year-old female on a 1200 kcal diet to lose 15 kg She weighs 85 kg, is 165 cm tall and is considered sedentary.

In this case we need to solve for the time (t) required to lose weight. Use equation 1.

where t time in days
     γ energy value per unit of mass, of body mass lost = 7700
     W_0 initial weight = 85 kg
     W_f final weight = 85 – 15 = 70 kg
     A age = 30 years
     Ka activity level = 8 kcal/kg/day (from Table 1 for sedentary)
     H height = 165 cm

For 30-year old female:

$$B = 6.25H - 4.92A - 161 = 6.25(165) - 4.92(30) - 161 = 722.7$$
$$K_1 = 0.9DI - B = 0.9(1200) - 722.7 = 1080 - 722.7 = 357.3 \,,$$
$$K_2 = Ka + 9.99 = 8.0 + 9.99 = 17.99$$

Substitute above values for all parameters into equation 1:

$$t = -\frac{\gamma}{K_2}\ln\left[\frac{K_1-K_2W_f}{K_1-K_2W_0}\right] = -\frac{7700}{17.99}\ln\left[\frac{357.3-17.99(70)}{357.3-17.99(85)}\right] = 112 \text{ days}$$

Example 2. Determine the dietary intake required for a 30-year old female to lose 15 kg in 100 days. She is 165 cm tall, weighs 90 kg and her activity level is thought to be light. From Table 1, $Ka = 10.0$. (This example is particularly useful for nutritionists and dieticians.)

In this case we need to solve for the dietary intake (DI) required to lose a given amount of weight and we use equation 2.

$K_2 = 10.0 + 9.99 = 19.99$, As in example 1, $B = 722.7$, $\gamma = 7700$, $\alpha = 0.10$ but $W_0 = 90$ kg, $W_f = 75$ kg and $t = 100$ days. Substitute these values into equation 2.

$$DI = \frac{(-19.99(90)-722.7)\exp\left\{-\dfrac{100(19.99)}{7700}\right\}+19.99(75)+722.7}{(\exp\left\{-\dfrac{100(19.99)}{7700}\right\}-1)(-1+0.10)} = 1345 \text{ kcal/d}$$

Thus this dieter should eat 1345 kcal per day to lose 15 kg in 100 days.

Example 3. How much weight will a 60-year old male on 1200 kcal diet lose in 100 days? He weighs 95 kg, is 178 cm tall and is considered moderately active.

For 60-year old male:

$B = 6.25H - 4.92A + 5 = 6.25(165) - 4.92(60) + 5 = 741.1$

$K_1 = 0.9DI - B = 0.9(1200) - 741.1 = 1080 - 741.1 = 338.9$

$Ka = 13.0$ (from Table 1 for moderately active)

$K_2 = Ka + 9.99 = 13.0 + 9.99 = 22.99$

In this case we need to solve for his final weight (W_f) after 100 days on a 1200 kcal diet. Use equation 3. Substitute the appropriate values into equation 3:

$$W_f = \frac{(22.99(95)-338.9)\exp\left(-\dfrac{100(22.99)}{7700}\right)+338.9}{22.99} = 74.3 \text{ kg}$$

134

Then the amount of weight this man would lose is given by equation 4:

$$\Delta W = W_0 - W_f = 95 - 74.3 = 20.7 \text{ kg}$$

Summary   The new Antonetti-Thomas weight loss predictive model provides a simple, straight-forward method to calculate realistic weight loss for an individual or at a population-wide level.

Appendix F Bibliography

1. Atwater and F.G. Benedict 1903 Experiments on the metabolism of matter and energy in the human body. U.S. Dept Agriculture Bull. 136.

2. Antonetti, V.W. 1973 The equations governing weight change in human beings. *Am J Clin Nutr* 26 (1):64-71.

3. Bruen, C. 1930 Variation of basal metabolic rate per unit surface area with age. *J Gen Physiol* 13 (6):607-610.

4. Antonetti, V.W. 1973 *The Computer Diet: A Weight Control Guide.* New York, M. Evans.

5. Mifflin, M.D., S.T. St. Jeor, et al. 1990 A new predictive equation for resting energy expenditure in healthy individuals. *J Clin Nutr* 51 (2):241.

6. Thomas, D.M. and V.W. Antonetti. Dynamic modeling of energy expenditure to estimate Dietary Energy Intake. from Schoeller, D.A. and M. Westerterp-Plantenga,ed. 2017 *Advances in the Assessment of Dietary Intake.* New York, CRC Press, Chapter 12: 211-219.

7. Westerterp, K.R., et al. 1995 Energy intake, physical activity and body weight: A simulation model. *Br J Nutr* 73 (3):337-347.

8. Hall, K.D. 2010 Predicting metabolic adaptation, body weight change, and energy intake in humans. *Am J Endrocrinol Metab* 298(3):E449-E466.

9. Thomas, D.M., et al. 2011 A simple model predicting weight change in humans. *J Bio Dyn* 5 (6):579-599.

10. Thomas, D.M., et al. 2014 Time to correctly predict the amount of weight loss with dieting. *J Acad Nutr Diet* 114 (6):857.

11. Taylor, C.M. and O.F. Pye. *Foundations of Nutrition.* New York, Macmillan, 1966, p. 48.

12. Moran, M.J., et al. *Fundamentals of Engineering Thermodynamics,* New York, Wiley, 2014.

NoPaperPress eBooks and Paperbacks

100-Day Super Diet-1200 Cal*
100-Day Super Diet-1500 Cal*
100-Day No-Cooking Diet-1200 Cal*
100-Day No-Cooking Diet-1500 Cal*
90-Day Smart Diet-1200 Cal*
90-Day Smart Diet-1500 Cal*
90-Day No-Cooking Diet - 1200 Cal*
90-Day No-Cooking Diet - 1500 Cal*
90-Day Perfect Diet - 1200 Cal*
90-Day Perfect Diet - 1500 Cal*
60-Day Perfect Diet-1200 Cal*
60-Day Perfect Diet-1500 Cal*
50-Day Flex Diet-1200 Cal*
50-Day Flex Diet-1500 Cal*
30-Day Quick Diet - Women*
30-Day Quick Diet for Men*
30-Day No-Cooking Diet*
30-Day Diet - Women - Metric*
30-Day Diet for Men - Metric*
25 Day Easy Diet-1200 Cal*
25 Day Easy Diet-1500 Cal*
25-Day No-Cooking Diet
10-Day Express Diet
10-Day No-Cooking Diet*
7-Day Diet for Women*
7-Day Diet for Men*
7-Day No-Cooking Diets*
90-Day Gluten-Free Diet-1200 Cal*
90-Day Gluten-Free Diet-1500 Cal*
30-Day Gluten-Free Quick Diet*
30-Day Gluten-Free No-Cooking Diet*
7-Day Diet for Women - Metric*
7-Day Diet for Men - Metric
7-Day Gluten-Free Express Diet*
7-Day Gluten-Free No-Cooking Diet*
90-Day Vegetarian Diet-1200 Cal*
90-Day Vegetarian Diet-1500 Cal*
30-Day Vegetarian Diet*
7-Day Vegetarian Diet*
Weight Loss for Women*
Weight Loss for Women - Metric
Weight Loss for Women - UK
Weight Loss for Men*
Maximum Weight Loss - 1200 Cal*
Maximum Weight Loss - 1500 Cal*

Weight Loss for Men - Metric*
Maximum Weight Loss- 1200 Cal*
Maximum Weight Loss- 1500 Cal*
Weight Control - U.S. Edition*
Weight Control - Metric. Edition
Prof Weight Control Women - U.S.
Prof Weight Control Women - Metric
Prof Weight Control Men - U.S.
Prof Weight Control Men - Metric
Weight Maintenance - U.S. Ed*
Weight Maintenance - Metric. Ed*
Weight Maintenance - UK Ed
Weight Loss for Senior Men*
Weight Loss for Senior Women*
Eat Smart - U.S. Edition*
Eat Smart - Metric Edition
30-Day Mediterranean Diet
Exercise Smart - U.S. Edition*
Exercise Smart - Metric Edition
Exercise Smart - UK Edition*
Total Fitness - U.S. Edition
Total Fitness - Metric Edition
Total Fitness - UK Edition
Total Fitness for Women-U.S. Ed*
Total Fitness for Women - Metric
Total Fitness for Women - UK Ed
Total Fitness for Men - U.S. Ed*
Total Fitness for Men- Metric Ed*
Total Fitness for Men - UK Ed
Senior Fitness - U.S. Edition*
Senior Fitness - Metric Edition*
Senior Fitness - UK Edition*
Computer Diet - U.S. Edition*
Computer Diet - Metric Ed*
Reliable Weight Loss - U.S. Ed
101 Weight Loss Tips*
101 Healthy Eating Tips*
101 Lifelong Fitness Tips*
101 Weight Maintenance Tips
101 Weight Loss Recipes
101 GF Weight Loss Recipes
101 Veggie Weight Loss Recipes*
30-Day Mediterranean Diet*
90-Day Mediterranean Diet - 1200 Cal*
90-Day Mediterranean Diet - 1500 Cal*

* These titles are available as both ebooks and paperbacks. Our ebooks are sold by Amazon, Apple, Google, Barnes & Noble and Kobo, but our paperbacks are only sold by Amazon.

Disclaimer

This book offers general weight control information. It is not a medical manual and the author does not claim to be medically qualified. The material in this book is not intended to be a substitute for medical counseling. Everyone should have a medical checkup before beginning a weight loss program. Moreover, the physician conducting the medical exam should be made aware of and should approve the specific weight control program planned. Additionally, while the author and publisher have made every effort to ensure the accuracy of the information in this book, they make no representations or warranties regarding its accuracy or completeness. Further, neither the author nor publisher assume liability for any medical problems that might result from applying the methods in this book, or for any loss of profit, or any other commercial damages, including but not limited to special, incidental, consequential or other damages, and any such liability is hereby expressly disclaimed.

Vincent W. Antonetti, Ph.D. is an emeritus professor at Manhattan College. He is a weight control and fitness expert who has lectured on

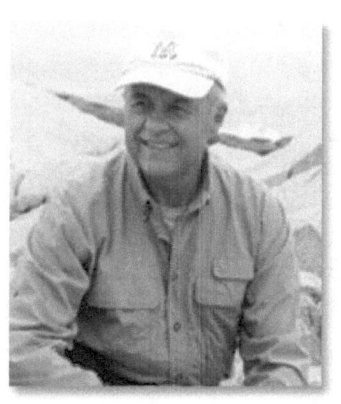

fitness at IBM Management and Professional Development classes and often speaks on fitness and weight control. Among his many publications is his highly regarded "The Equations Governing Weight Change in Human Beings," published in the prestigious American Journal of Clinical Nutrition. This paper was the first to develop an accurate equation to calculate weight loss. Dr. Antonetti's critically acclaimed book *The Computer Diet* was given Consumer Guide magazine's highest recommendation. Recently, Dr. Antonetti coauthored "A Computational Tool to Simulate Energy Balance Components in Pharmacological Interventions," presented at Obesity Week 2016. He also co-authored (with Professor Diana Thomas) "Dynamic Modeling of Energy Expenditure to Estimate Dietary Energy Intake," Chapter 12 in Advances in the Assessment of Dietary Intake, published July 2017 by CRC Press. He is also the author or co-author of more than 100 eBooks and paperbacks. Most of Dr. Antonetti's books are listed at: www.nopaperpress.com.

Professor Antonetti is a life long exercise and nutrition enthusiast. Although a senior citizen he still maintains a vigorous physical fitness program - and has managed to maintain his weight to within 2 lbs (about one kg) of the 154 lbs (70 kg) it was when he graduated from college many years ago. He is now semi-retired and living in The Villages, Florida.